Who's in Charge?

WHO'S IN CHARGE?

Leadership during Epidemics, Bioterror
Attacks, and other Public Health Crises

Laura H. Kahn

PRAEGER SECURITY INTERNATIONAL
An Imprint of ABC-CLIO, LLC

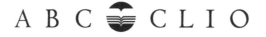

A B C CLIO

Santa Barbara, California • Denver, Colorado • Oxford, England

Library of Congress Cataloging-in-Publication Data

Kahn, Laura H.
   Who's in charge : leadership during epidemics, bioterror attacks, and other public
health crises / Laura H. Kahn.
       p. cm.
   Includes bibliographical references and index.
   ISBN 978-0-275-99485-3 (hardcover : alk. paper)—ISBN 978-1-56720-760-6 (ebook)
1. Public health administration—United States.   2. Public health—United States.
3. Leadership.   I. Title.
   RA445.K24   2009
   362.1—dc22   2009022273

13   12   11   10   09   1   2   3   4   5

This book is also available on the World Wide Web as an eBook.
Visit www.abc-clio.com for details.

ABC-CLIO, LLC
130 Cremona Drive, P.O. Box 1911
Santa Barbara, California 93116-1911

This book is printed on acid-free paper ∞
Manufactured in the United States of America

CONTENTS

ACKNOWLEDGMENTS

This book would not have been possible without the help of many people—elected officials, physicians, veterinarians, public health and hospital officials, law enforcement officials, journalists, and scientists—who took the time to share their experiences and opinions with me: Sir Roy Anderson, Joseph Annelli, Donald Behm, Georges Benjamin, Ruth Berkelman, Larry Bush, Isabelle Chmitelin, Neil Cohen, George DiFerdinando, Alex Donaldson, Mark Ghilarducci, Glen Gilmore, Kevin Hayden, D. A. Henderson, Bonnie Henry, Bill Jobes, Larry Kerr, Paul Kitching, Jeff Koplan, Lord John Krebs, Donald Low, Lord John MacGregor, Hugh Mainzer, Jean Marie Malecki, Jean-Claude Manuguerra, Lord Robert May, Keith Meldrum, Thomas Monath, Paul Nannis, John Norquist, Case Ootes, Joseph Palma, Daksh Patel, Mark Perkiss, Andre Picard, Irwin Redlener, Richard Schabas, David Sencer, Kenneth Shuey, Alan Sipress, Karen Sliter, Christy Stephenson, Thomas Taft, Maureen Taylor, and Alex Thiermann.

I am extremely grateful to those who provided invaluable advice, comments, criticisms, references, suggestions, or other forms of assistance: Sir Donald Acheson, David Ashford, Jeremiah Barondess, Richard Besser, Guthrie Birkhead, Chris Chyba, Leonard Cole, Lisa Conti, Gill Dilmitis, Andrew Flacks, Zachary Fink, David Fisman, Sheldon Garon, Paul Gibbs, Fred Greenstein, Elin Gursky, Saskia Hendrickx, William Hueston, Robert Kahn, Bruce Kaplan, Richard Keevey, Barbara Kellerman, Nannerl Keohane, Lonnie King, Eric and Jeff Kutner, Stephen Leeder, Caroline Moreau, Gerald Parker, Richard Preston, Stuart Rabner, Barbara Reynolds, Michele Russell, Mark Scheibner, James Steele, James Weed, and Kerr White.

I would like to thank Suzanne Staszak-Silva, formerly at Praeger Security International, for approaching me to write this book. I would like to thank Ezra Suleiman for introducing me to the writings of Max Weber. Linda Benson, Timothy Ryan, and Darryl Taylor provided invaluable editorial assistance. Finally, I would not have been able to write this book without the love and support of my husband, David Spergel, and my children, Julian, Sarah, and Joshua.

Chapter 1

UNDERSTANDING LEADERSHIP

AN OVERVIEW OF LEADERSHIP

Leadership is critical for responding to disease crises. Whether an epidemic spreads naturally or through bioterrorism, any crisis can pose difficult challenges for leaders. Novel pathogens, such as the avian influenza or Severe Acute Respiratory Syndrome (SARS) virus, are particularly problematic because of the initial absence of scientific information about them. Leaders might need input from physicians, veterinarians, public health officials, scientists, economists, lawyers, and ethicists to make effective decisions.

Even with such expert advice, officials might not fully anticipate the implications of various response policies. For example, people's economic interests might lead them to oppose neighborhood quarantines, food bans, or the slaughter of livestock. In some severe cases, policies can have unintended consequences, such as protest demonstrations and suicides. For example, during the 2001 foot-and-mouth disease crisis in the United Kingdom, veterinarians protested the cruel livestock-slaughtering policies, and some farmers committed suicide because they were overwhelmed by the loss of their herds.[1]

Officials might not fully understand their own roles and responsibilities if these have not been clearly articulated in public health or disaster response laws, policies, or procedures. In the United States, leadership is decentralized and crisis responses are primarily state and local government responsibilities. States vary considerably in their public health laws, but the role of the federal government is primarily supportive. In countries such as the United Kingdom, the national government is more directly involved.[2]

Individual personalities might come into play during crises: some elected officials might prefer to delegate decision making, whereas others might prefer to make all of the decisions themselves. In either case, if those responsible do not take charge or do so ineffectually, a leadership vacuum results, leading to turf battles, leadership confusion, and response delays.

The decision to mass vaccinate a human population during an epidemic might be a political one; however, the public may balk, on the theory that such decisions are politically motivated. Prior to the invasion of Iraq in 2003, President George W. Bush's mass smallpox vaccination program for first responders turned into a debacle because it was viewed as a purely political decision because there was no medical indication for vaccination.[3] The smallpox threat was hypothetical since the disease had been eradicated from human populations in 1977. The medical community was skeptical because it did not know the risks versus the benefits of such a program.[4] Many people developed adverse reactions to the vaccine, and one person died from an acute myocardial infarction after receiving it.[5] Ultimately, the smallpox threat never materialized.[6]

STUDYING PUBLIC HEALTH LEADERSHIP

Numerous reports, papers, books, and exercises have addressed the nature of public health leadership and many recommend that leadership roles and responsibilities be better specified. Some identify the qualities needed for good leadership and recommend teaching officials how to be better leaders. Tabletop exercises, which simulate crises and provide practice opportunities for government officials, have identified leadership problems that can arise during crises. This book explores *why* leadership problems develop during disease outbreaks.

In 1988, the Institute of Medicine (IOM) published *The Future of Public Health,* written partly in response to a severe decline in support and funding for public health that began in 1981.[7] The public health infrastructure had been allowed to fall into disarray. The IOM report noted the tension that existed between politicians and professional experts throughout the nations' public health system.[8] Decisions were largely made in response to crises and were based primarily on competition, influence, and bargaining, rather than on comprehensive scientific analyses. In other words, public health agencies were not neutral and expert but, rather, highly political, and they have managed poorly with this reality.[9]

The rapid turnover of public health leaders, with tenures averaging only two years, supports this premise.[10] Indeed, few highly qualified individuals serve as leaders in public health agencies.[11] In addition, state boards of health used to exist in almost all the states but dwindled to only 24 since 1980.[12]

The report found that large numbers of public health personnel were not adequately prepared for their jobs. Schools of public health have traditionally focused their efforts on research and education, and not necessarily on the preparation of leaders to handle the conflicts between political forces and competing societal values.[13] The IOM report recommended, among other things, that public health leaders possess a wide range of capabilities, including scientific expertise; communication skills; managerial abilities; decision-making skills; mobilizing expertise for collective action; and, perhaps most important, skills in handling the political realities of government service.[14]

Fifteen years later, in 2003, the IOM revisited the status of public health in *The Future of the Public's Health in the 21st Century.*[15] The new report found a few successes in the area of public health leadership, such as the initiation of national and regional Public Health Leadership Institutes by the Centers for Disease Control and Prevention in 1992. However, the report found that many of the fundamental problems that have plagued the public health infrastructure, namely limited political and financial support (other than funding for bioterrorism), continued to persist. Many in the public health workforce still lacked basic competencies to help them meet routine and emergent challenges.

The 2003 report also noted that even though many individuals in public health had received leadership training at the national level, recruiting and retaining these individuals in leadership positions continued to be a major concern. Tenure for public health leaders, particularly for political appointees, remained short term, and political factors continued to play a major role in the ability, or inability, of public health leaders to influence policy.[16] The report recommended that leadership training, support, and development should be a high priority for government public health agencies and for schools of public health, and that competency in communication should be a critical core requirement for public health leaders.

The Public Health Leadership Institutes emphasize collaborative and team-based approaches to leadership in their training. One program initially accepted only teams, rather than individuals.[17] Educational modules include leadership style assessments, personal feedback and coaching, and team projects. The emphasis is on developing and strengthening cross-agency coalitions, consensus goals, and communications. However, topics such as understanding the relationships between elected officials and public health professionals, the politics of decision making, or the reasons that leadership problems develop during crises are not specifically mentioned.

Trust for America's Health, a nonprofit organization that measures public health quality indicators, has been publishing annual reports on the state of public health emergency preparedness in the United States since 2003.[18] In its 2008 report, based on data collected the previous year, the authors indicate that public health preparedness gains had been made after nearly $1 billion was allocated annually to states since the passage of the Public Health Security and Bioterrorism Act of 2002. However, according to the report, federal spending cuts of 25 percent to state and local preparedness efforts since 2005 could jeopardize that progress. The criteria used to measure state readiness focused on the acquisition of vaccines, availability of hospital beds, laboratory and surveillance capabilities, laws to limit medical volunteer liability, and funding for public health services. The report stated that two ongoing key areas of concern were leadership and accountability and recommended that leadership roles and responsibilities should be clarified at the federal level.[19]

Tabletop exercises assessing capabilities during simulated bioterrorist attacks also uncovered leadership problems. In June 2001, the Johns Hopkins Center for Civilian Biodefense Strategies, in collaboration with the Oklahoma National Memorial Institute for the Prevention of Terrorism, the Center for Strategic and International Studies (CSIS), and the Analytic Services Institute for Homeland Security (ANSER), conducted a simulated bioterrorist attack called "Dark Winter" with 12 federal and state senior-level politicians who portrayed members of the National Security Council.[20] The exercise presented a fictional scenario, a covert smallpox attack that required participants to establish strategies and make policy response decisions. The senior-level politicians included Sam Nunn, the former U.S. senator from Georgia, who played the president of the United States, and Frank Keating, the governor of Oklahoma, who played himself. The goal of the exercise was to examine the challenges that senior policymakers would face if confronted with a bioterrorist attack, and to increase their awareness of the unique difficulties such a crisis would present. The scenario involved three separate attacks in shopping malls in Oklahoma City, Oklahoma; Atlanta, Georgia; and Philadelphia, Pennsylvania.

The total number of smallpox cases in the exercise swelled to 30,000, of which approximately one-third died. The authors of the exercise estimated that in a worst case scenario, the epidemic would progress to include as many as 3 million cases with 1 million deaths. The vaccine supply was limited and dwindling, and new vaccine would not be available for at least a month.

The terrorists were threatening more attacks. The scenario ended with the senior-level policymakers faced not only with a spreading deadly infectious disease, but also with a national security crisis. Analysts concluded that the senior-level politicians were unfamiliar with the policy implications of such a public health crisis and would be highly dependent on accurate data, which might not be available, and on the expertise of medical and public health professionals to deal with the infectious disease.[21]

Leadership problems also surfaced in another tabletop exercise called "TOPOFF," for "Top Official." In May 2000, the U.S. Department of Justice conducted the $3-million "TOPOFF" drill to test the preparedness of senior-level government officials for terrorist attacks in Portsmouth, New Hampshire; Washington, D.C.; and Denver, Colorado. Only Denver experienced a simulated bioterrorist attack. The other two cities dealt with either chemical or radiological terrorism.

In Denver, the exercise scenario involved the covert release of the plague bacteria *Yersinia pestis* at the Denver Performing Arts Center. Participants included officials from the state and county health agencies, the Centers for Disease Control and Prevention, the Public Health Service, the Office of Emergency Preparedness, and three local hospitals. The governor of Colorado did not participate; instead simulated decisions were made. As the number of sick and dying increased, the simulated governor commandeered all antibiotics that could be used to prevent or treat plague and issued an executive order to restrict all travel into or out of the city. Despite these efforts, the outbreak spread to other states, as well as to England and Japan. The exercise ended with reports estimating 3,060 to more than 4,000 individuals sick with plague in the United States and abroad, with 800 to more than 2,000 deaths. The scenario closed with civil unrest and riots.[22]

One of the major findings of TOPOFF was confusion regarding leadership, the role of the authorities, and the decision-making processes. Since the governor of Colorado, Bill Owens, did not participate in the exercise, the decision-making authority was transferred to the governor's Emergency Epidemic Response Committee, which usually serves as an advisory committee to the governor. Indeed, in the absence of the governor, or an alternative elected official with legal authority, the committee, by law, did not have the legal authority to make decisions. Nevertheless, it did make decisions.

These decisions were made by conference calls and were fraught with serious difficulties and delays. Disagreements among the participants were common and decisions were frequently reversed. In addition, a variety of state and federal emergency management and law enforcement agencies set up emergency operations centers, which added to the leadership confusion. Communication systems were chaotic. One conclusion of the exercise was that political leadership is essential to manage a public health crisis. Without such leadership, there would be no moral and legal authority to enact potentially controversial decisions. In addition, scientific experts are needed to serve as advisors to the politicians.[23]

These efforts highlight some of the leadership problems that can develop during crises, but they do not explain why the problems arise in the first place. In this book, five disease crises undergo intensive analyses. Newspaper articles, books, government inquiries, and medical literature were reviewed to provide a chronological account of the outbreaks. In addition, elected officials, public health professionals, physicians, veterinarians, scientists, journalists, and law enforcement officials were interviewed to provide insight into individual experiences during the crises. The goal is to delve deeply into each crisis, to gather many different points of view, and to recreate as complete a picture as possible as to what actually happened and why.

POLITICAL LEADERS AND BUREAUCRATS

At the turn of the 20th century, Max Weber, the German sociologist, wrote that an inherent conflict of interest exists between elected and bureaucratic leaders. Specifically, elected leaders strive to get reelected and implement their ideologically based policies, whereas bureaucratic leaders aim to perpetuate and expand their bureaucracies.[24] Weber's theories on political power and bureaucracies are relevant to understanding crisis leadership because the inherent structure of democracies and their constitutional frameworks influence how elected officials and bureaucratic leaders work together. Bureaucratic leaders must necessarily be highly trained experts in their respective fields; elected leaders must collaborate with them without losing dominance. During any crisis, therefore, there are at least two leaders: the elected leader and the bureaucratic leader.

At the federal level, one could argue that there are at least three leaders. For example, President Bush appointed Tommy Thompson, a former governor of Wisconsin, to be secretary of Health and Human Services in 2001. Dr. Jeffrey Koplan, appointed by former President Bill Clinton, was director of the Centers for Disease Control and Prevention. During the 2001 anthrax crisis, Dr. Koplan and his staff were accused of being inaccessible and of not providing enough information to the public. The situation worsened when Thompson went before the press and gave medical information that many believed should have come from Dr. Koplan.[25] In this example, there were three leaders: President Bush, Tommy Thompson, and Jeffrey Koplan.

President Bush's managerial style may have contributed to the perception that the government was not in control of the situation. Bush was portrayed as being a hands-off chief executive who preferred to delegate all tasks. He had less government experience than anyone in his cabinet,[26] and his lack of experience and tendency to delegate may have set the stage for a series of power struggles among the top bureaucratic appointees. Dr. Koplan announced his resignation on February 22, 2002—six months after the anthrax letters were first mailed.[27] Koplan appeared to be the scapegoat for a poorly coordinated and articulated government response to the bioterrorist attacks.

It is important to keep in mind, however, that the relationship between elected and bureaucratic leaders may differ from one democracy to another depending on their respective constitutional frameworks and how the bureaucratic leaders obtain their positions, as the following examples show.[28] In the United States, the elected leader is responsible for appointing people who, theoretically at least,[29] have the specialized education and expertise to administer and manage an emergency response through the bureaucracy. At the highest levels of government, the U.S. president and others within the executive branch have access to scientific experts. For example, the National Science Policy and Organization Act of 1975 established the Office of Science and Technology Policy in 1976 to provide advice on scientific and technology questions relevant to national and international issues. The U.S. Office of Technology Assessment provided members of the U.S. Congress with analysis of highly technical and scientific issues for 23 years (1972–95); however, its funding was withdrawn by Congress in 1995. Such expert advice might not be available for other elected officials, particularly at the local level.

In France, the placement of bureaucratic leaders follows the model of ancient China with a system of education for the future elite. France has a highly selective and competitive university, the École Nationale d'Administration, from which the best and the brightest get the top jobs—in both politics and the nation's highly centralized bureaucracy. Thus, relationships in France are fluid because bureaucratic leaders can easily become elected leaders.[30]

In contrast to both the U.S. and French systems, bureaucrats in the United Kingdom (UK) are usually secure in their positions, whereas politicians come and go from office more frequently.[31] The higher-level civil servants in the UK are placed after careful selection and cultivation over many years; they are, in essence, socialized for their positions, and they provide institutional memory within their departments. This system was established in 1854 by the Northcote-Trevelyan Commission, which recommended the creation of a civil service that was based on merit rather than on personal or party connections or nepotism.[32]

This concept of multiple leaders also applies to nondemocratically elected governments such as that of China, but possibly to a lesser extent.

In such governments, political leaders still depend on bureaucrats to carry out their policies, but they may be less accountable for poorly managed government actions because they have not been elected by the people, and the bureaucratic leaders may not have been appointed by the leaders currently in power.

DEFINING LEADERSHIP

An important step in understanding why leadership problems arise during crises is to review what is known about leaders and leadership. Questions about leaders and leadership have intrigued scholars in both Western and Eastern civilizations for centuries. Plato, Confucius, and Machiavelli all speculated about leaders, and even though they lived in different eras and different places, they did seem to agree that leaders should possess knowledge, wisdom, and ability. They should lead by example and demonstrate moral and ethical behavior to retain their power and position.

Although ancient philosophers described the qualities necessary for leaders, they did not define leadership itself. According to James MacGregor Burns, leadership is one of the most observed, yet least understood, phenomena on our planet.[33] Burns defined two types of leadership: transactional and transforming. *Transactional leadership* is the more common: leaders approach followers with goals of exchanging one thing for another. For example, elected leaders seek votes in exchange for jobs or campaign contributions in exchange for subsidies.

In contrast, *transforming leadership* is more complex and powerful. Rather than simply an exchange of goods or services, transforming leadership occurs when a leader engages followers to seek higher levels of motivation, morality, and/or purpose. This type of leadership is unequivocally linked to followers' needs and goals. Power certainly has a role here; however, leaders use their power to motivate people, not to treat them as objects.[34]

The ability to motivate organizations such as government bureaucracies to respond to crises would probably fall under the category of transforming leadership. Unfortunately, in general, bureaucracies have not had a stellar reputation of responding to societies' needs but rather respond to their own. As Burns writes, "Too often bureaucracies acknowledge only their internal reciprocity and the transactional relationship between managers and employees and in consequence respond to their own mutual wants, needs, motives, and values without acknowledging the primary relationship, which is external."[35]

In essence, a leader is someone who can make something happen that would not happen otherwise.[36] This definition applies to the head of any group of people, from a small family or tribe to a large organization or a government.[37] It applies to both elected and appointed (bureaucratic) leaders. It applies to leaders of nongovernment organizations and businesses that may participate in crisis responses, although they would ultimately not be held responsible for the outcomes.

This book examines leadership, particularly the relationship between elected and appointed officials, during disease crises. After a brief historical overview of public health and bioterrorism in chapters 2 and 3, political leadership, public health leadership, and communication skills are explored in depth in chapters 4, 5, and 8 by studying three cases: the 2001 anthrax attacks in several U.S. states; the 1993 cryptosporidium outbreak in Milwaukee, Wisconsin; and the 2003 SARS outbreak in Toronto, Canada.

Since many newly emerging infectious diseases infecting humans come from animals, chapters 6 and 7 explore leadership during the scientific uncertainty that often accompanies animal health crises. New diseases that involve animals, such as bovine spongiform encephalopathy (BSE), also known as "mad cow" disease, are particularly difficult to respond to because often it is not known if the disease can infect humans. In the case of BSE, almost a decade passed before human cases were identified. Other diseases, such as foot-and-mouth disease, infect only animals but indirectly affect humans in profound ways.

Chapter 9 explores worst case scenarios: when crises overwhelm local capabilities and disrupt normal societal functioning, such as the 1918–19 influenza pandemic. The legal challenges to public health during bioterrorist attacks are discussed, as well as the roles and responsibilities of law enforcement, emergency management, public health, and the military. A bioterrorist attack is both an attack against the national security of a country and a public health crisis.

Who is in charge during a crisis can have an enormous impact on how many lives are saved or lost. Leaders must make decisions and communicate them effectively to many different groups. Understanding how this process works, and how it can go wrong, should help future political leaders, public and animal health leaders, media professionals, and the public better prepare for the disease crises they may face.

Chapter 2

THE LONG MARCH TO IMPROVING THE PUBLIC'S HEALTH

In 1798, an outbreak of yellow fever in New York City killed nearly 2,000 people. A committee was convened to investigate the epidemic, but it would be almost a year before it delivered its recommendations. The committee called for better sanitation to halt the epidemic and for the city government to regulate the construction and condition of all toilets, inspect all buildings and grounds, and clean the streets. Despite these recommendations, sanitary conditions worsened in the following years.[1]

Yellow fever epidemics had been sweeping the East Coast of the United States since 1791. This deadly viral illness transmitted by mosquitoes caused thousands to die in Boston, New York City, and Philadelphia. Yet with each new outbreak, the initial response of city leaders was to panic, not to execute carefully prepared public health plans. Worse, leaders did not learn from the experiences of others: although well aware of the 1798 yellow fever outbreak in New York City, Boston did not establish a board of health until a year later, after a severe yellow fever epidemic killed nearly 300 people in that city.[2]

It would be ideal if leaders could foresee crises and plan their responses in advance. But throughout most of human history, this has been seldom the case. However, beginning in the 18th century, leaders in medicine, science, and law started making significant discoveries and contributions in public health. Some endured personal ridicule, criticism, and threats for their novel ideas. In many cases, these leaders succeeded in saving lives despite initial opposition to their efforts.

INFECTIOUS DISEASE EPIDEMICS

Infectious diseases, such as smallpox, plague, cholera, malaria, yellow fever, and influenza, have afflicted humans throughout the ages and have caused untold suffering and death.[3] During the mid-14th century, nearly a third of the population of Europe died from plague, also called the Black Death.[4] Such infectious diseases have altered the course of history, wiping out leaders, armies, kingdoms, and sometimes entire civilizations.[5] Old World diseases, such as smallpox, arrived with the Europeans in the Western Hemisphere and killed large numbers of the susceptible Native American populations.[6] Sometimes diseases, particularly smallpox and plague, were spread deliberately through biowarfare (see chapter 3).[7]

An infectious disease epidemic emerges when many people (or animals) become infected with a pathogen.[8] When humans abandoned their hunting and gathering lifestyle for a sedentary, but more secure and productive, life of agriculture, they inadvertently created the perfect conditions for epidemics.[9] Bacteria, viruses, protozoa, and other infectious microorganisms require a concentration of susceptible hosts to set off and propagate an infectious disease epidemic.

The small farming communities that humans settled into soon grew into villages, towns, and cities, densely packed with people. Human waste was not properly disposed of, and clean water was not available. New agriculture methods concentrated crops and irrigation canals and domesticated livestock, decreasing biodiversity and increasing the risk of disease. Humans and animals lived close to one another, sometimes even sharing living quarters.[10]

For much of history, however, ancient peoples did not attribute infectious disease epidemics to natural causes; instead, they believed sickness was divine retribution for immoral behavior (the Israelites), the wrath of mythological beings or bad air miasmas (the Greeks), and demons and spirits (pre-Islamic Arabs), among other explanations.[11]

Some ancient societies began to recognize that epidemics were a part of nature, and that their harm could be minimized, if not eliminated altogether, through better sanitation. Sewage and foul water were linked to illness. Hippocrates (ca. 460 BCE–ca. 370 BCE), the famous Greek physician, wrote "Airs, Waters, and Places" and promoted the concept of public health through a clean environment.[12] Starting in 312 BCE, the Romans created extensive aqueduct systems to bring clean water into their cities and built latrines for public use.[13]

Sanitation practices declined precipitously during the Middle Ages, however, as rational approaches to health were replaced by religious beliefs. There was little incentive to improve public health if epidemics were considered a test of the faithful.[14] Still, some lessons that had been learned continued to be practiced. People understood that sick people and corpses should be kept isolated and away from the healthy; ships containing people ill with the plague were often quarantined in an attempt to prevent the spread of disease. When the Black Death was raging in the Middle Ages, some civil and medical authorities wrote ordinances that corpses should be buried in trenches six to eight feet deep.[15]

Nearly all of these practices were based on instinct, folklore, and old wives' tales, rather than on evidence. It would be many years before scientists would systematically study the causes and methods of controlling infectious diseases.

Europeans initiated the idea of collecting population data for analysis and policy development in the mid-17th century. The Englishman William Petty (1623–87), a physician and economist, invented the term *political arithmetic* to describe the collection of population data.[16] John Graunt (1620–74) took Petty's ideas and wrote his famous book *Natural and Political Observations Made upon the Bills of Mortality,* in which he analyzed deaths in London from the preceding third of a century with simple statistics. He showed that even imperfect data, if carefully analyzed and interpreted, could provide useful information. Unfortunately, the English Civil War in the mid-17th century ended any efforts to use political arithmetic to improve public health until the passage of the Poor Laws 170 years later.[17]

VACCINES: A FORTUNATE COINCIDENCE

Smallpox is believed to have appeared in the first agricultural settlements in northeastern Africa around 10,000 BCE. Egyptian merchants then carried it to India and Asia. The virus, which eventually spread around the world, killed more people than any other microorganism throughout history.[18]

Possibly as early as the 10th century in China, people began to recognize that individuals who survived smallpox were immune to the disease for the rest of their lives. In an attempt to transfer this immunity to others, people would inoculate someone never previously infected with the disease with the pus-like material from a recovering individual's body.[19] This material would either be inserted into the person's nostrils or scratched into the skin with a lancet in the hope that the individual would get a mild form of smallpox, survive, and become immune.

Lady Mary Wortley Montagu, the wife of the British ambassador to Turkey, introduced this practice to Europe in the 18th century. After observing its effectiveness on children in the Ottoman Empire, Lady Montagu had it performed on her son in 1718, and in 1721, during a severe smallpox epidemic in England, on her four-year-old daughter. Both children survived. With time, despite deaths from the practice itself, which deliberately infected people with smallpox, acceptance spread throughout England.[20] In 1754, the Royal College of Physicians gave its official approval to the procedure.

In the late 18th century, a physician's apprentice, Edward Jenner, heard a country girl say that she would never get smallpox because she had already had cowpox.[21] Her statement reflected a common belief, and Jenner decided to test this folklore. Instead of inoculating patients using smallpox pus, he would use cowpox pus.

In May 1796, Jenner scratched cowpox pus from Sarah Nelmes, a milkmaid who developed cowpox on her hands after milking a cow, into the arm of eight-year-old James Phipps, his gardener's son. The boy became immune to smallpox. Jenner repeated the experiment on 13 others, and they also became immune.

In what would become a recurring theme throughout the history of medicine and public health, Jenner's ideas were initially criticized and his reputation threatened by established physicians before ultimately being accepted. Jenner sent a manuscript describing his results to the Philosophical Transactions of the Royal Society, which rejected his paper and warned him that he should never propose such an idea again if he valued his reputation. Jenner self-published his work and in the process created the terms *vaccination* and *vaccines,* derived from the Latin for cow, *vaca.* The paper was initially met with severe criticism, but acceptance eventually spread.

Although it would take a century to understand why vaccination induces immunity, Jenner's discovery was one of the greatest advances in medicine, and it changed the course of history. In 1980, after a decade-long, intensive worldwide vaccination campaign, the World Health Organization declared smallpox eradicated from human populations.

AN UNFORTUNATE SIDE EFFECT OF HOSPITALS

Prior to the 18th century, patients were treated in their homes, not in hospitals. Physicians established lying-in hospitals in the mid-18th century primarily to provide training opportunities for medical students in obstetrics, particularly in the use of forceps. The unintended consequence of these hospitals was the spread of puerperal, or childbirth, fever. Puerperal fever was caused by the bacteria *Streptoccocus pyogenes,* which is the same bacteria that causes strep throat, impetigo, and toxic shock syndrome.[22]

At the time, there were two predominant theories for the cause of puerperal fever: inflammation or putrefaction. The physicians who believed that the disease was due to inflammation, an abnormal condition of the blood and circulatory system, proposed that the best course of treatment was copious bleeding. Those who believed that it was caused by putrefaction, a breakdown of living matter into dangerous airborne particles called putrid effluvium, believed that treatment should center on protecting the body from possible exposure by closing all the windows and covering up the patient with bedclothes.[23]

From 1772 to 1795, British physicians published a series of reports hypothesizing that puerperal fever was contagious and that the spread could be controlled. They supported the putrefaction theory: a filthy environment with foul air contributed to disease spread.[24] Still, it would be a century before there was a breakthrough in understanding the transmission of the disease. When the breakthrough occurred, it would happen under similar circumstances and on two different continents. These events are described later in this chapter under "Awakenings."

EARLY PUBLIC HEALTH EPIDEMICS IN THE NEWLY FORMED UNITED STATES

While physicians in Europe contended with a variety of diseases and epidemics, their counterparts in the United States were busy doing the same. From 1791 to 1822, concern about yellow fever epidemics swept the East Coast. In Philadelphia, an outbreak in August 1793 caused panic as townspeople, including most of the federal, state, and local officials, fled the city. Matthew Clarkson, the mayor of Philadelphia, stayed and took charge despite limited funds and resources. He borrowed money; recruited volunteers; and led them to arrange for the care of the sick, poor, and orphaned.[25]

Fearful that the epidemic in Philadelphia would spread, New York City implemented a strict quarantine, scaled up its sanitation efforts, and established a volunteer health committee. New York City's health officer inspected incoming ships, and the health committee broke all communication with Philadelphia.

Still, in 1795, a yellow fever epidemic emerged in New York City. The health committee took charge of Bellevue Hospital and established the policy that physicians should report all patients they suspected of having yellow fever, so that they could be taken to Bellevue. Many of the physicians did not cooperate with this policy because they did not agree with it: many correctly believed that yellow fever was not contagious.[26] Dr. Charles Buxton, secretary of the College of Physicians, defended the actions of these physicians, claiming that the removal of yellow fever patients to Bellevue was harmful to the patient; distressing to friends; needlessly alarming to the public; and, tellingly, resented by the doctors who objected to being dictated to.[27]

The New York Medical Society passed a resolution in 1796 insisting that the city clean up the streets and waterfront to prevent further epidemics.

That same year, the state legislature passed a law that established the New York City Health Office, which consisted of several appointed health commissioners, including a practicing physician to serve as health officer, with the authority to inspect ships, enforce quarantine, and implement sanitary ordinances. Though promising, these changes did not halt the epidemic. In 1798, nearly 2,000 more people died.

Boston also suffered from yellow fever epidemics, despite rigid harbor quarantine enforcement. In 1797, the General Court of Massachusetts gave municipalities the authority to appoint health officers and to enact limited sanitary measures and, in 1799, a Boston Board of Health was established after a severe yellow fever epidemic killed almost 300 people.[28]

According to John Duffy, the public health historian, efforts to improve public health in the United States languished from colonial times until before the Civil War largely because of an emphasis on individual rather than community health. The medical profession had little to offer in the way of prevention or treatment of diseases and received little respect.[29]

SWEEPING SOCIAL CHANGES IN EUROPE

It was the French Revolution, and the tremendous social upheavals it brought, that created fertile ground for improved sanitation and public health in Europe. The French developed the notion that scientists and physicians should serve as expert advisors to the state, and, as a result, the government would be better able to provide an improved quality of life to its citizens.[30]

Louis-René Villermé (1782–1863), an 1814 graduate of the newly founded Ecole de Médecine in Paris and an army surgeon during the Napoleonic wars, devoted his career to studying how society could improve the lives of its members.[31] He conducted hygienic and statistical studies for the Société Medicale d'Emulation and later for the prestigious Royal Academy of Medicine.

The Royal Academy promoted the idea of applying the scientific method to understanding epidemic disease. Paris and its inhabitants became Villermé's patients, from whom he and his fellow hygienists (scientists who promoted sanitation—clean water and the removal of wastes) collected, analyzed, and generalized public health data. Villermé cemented his reputation as a leader in the application of numerical reasoning to public health problems in 1828. His report, *Recherches statistiques sur la ville de Paris et le département de la Seine,* presumed a connection between economic status and mortality. Villermé subsequently published dozens of studies in which he used birth and death rates as primary indicators of social well-being or distress. Villermé was only one of several pioneers in public health during the French hygienic movement. Dr. Alexandre Parent-Duchâtelet (1790–1835) devoted most of his medical career to public health, publishing 29 articles on the subject, often collaborating with Villermé. Known internationally as the leading French urban and occupational hygienist, he was a principal spokesperson for the new specialty of public hygiene and was largely responsible for transforming the Paris health council—traditionally an advisory board to the prefect of police—into a bona fide public health institution.[32]

It was in the early 19th century that Jeremy Bentham (1748–1832), impressed by the French efforts at social reform, ushered through the British Parliament a set of "Poor Laws" that sought to provide relief for the indigent.[33] Edwin Chadwick, who was aware of Villermé's and Parent-Duchâtelet's work, was appointed to investigate how well these Poor Laws were administered.[34] Chadwick discovered many problems during his investigation and wrote a report with his economist colleague, Nassau Senior, in which he made a number of recommendations, including the need for centralization, uniformity, and efficiency. In 1834, the Poor Laws were amended, incorporating nearly all of the recommendations Chadwick had made in his report. The Poor Laws made the state responsible for public health and sanitation. The reasoning behind this was that keeping people healthy through sanitation would provide labor for newly developing industries and in the long run would save money.

The sanitary conditions of the rapidly growing factory towns in Great Britain were deplorable and mortality rates were rising. The New Poor Laws were instrumental in turning human labor into a commodity for the growing market economy of the Industrial Revolution. However, it was not until a deadly cholera epidemic hit England in 1832 and killed almost 22,000 people that public health reform began.[35]

Liverpool was arguably the worst city in England in terms of poor sanitation and overcrowding and was hardest hit by cholera.[36] The disease caused miserable deaths from profuse watery diarrhea, severe abdominal pain, and muscle cramps. Previously healthy individuals died in a day. More than 1,500 out of almost 5,000 with the disease died; the epidemic sparked eight major riots in the streets. Deaths from cholera and other epidemics of typhoid and typhus, as well as from relapsing fevers, caused severe economic and social losses. The stimulus for change was reaching a tipping point.

In 1839, Parliament instructed the Poor Law Commission to investigate the health of the English, Scottish, and Welsh working populations. Three years later, Chadwick produced a three-volume report emphasizing that filthy environmental conditions, including lack of drainage, piles of sewage, and unclean water, led to disease and death.[37] In essence, the report justified the growing sanitation movement to improve the public's health.

However, it took a deadly cholera epidemic in 1848 and intensive advocacy efforts by prominent individuals to motivate Parliament to approve a Public Health Act and establish a General Board of Health, empowered to establish local boards of health. The act gave local boards of health the authority to oversee sewage removal and water supplies and to appoint a medical officer of health who was required to be a legally qualified physician with skills in inspecting nuisances (defined as any act or condition that interferes with the well-being of others). In 1854, opponents' outcries against the General Board of Health's sanitation efforts reached such intensity that Parliament did not renew the Public Health Act and the General Board of Health came to an end; however, the seeds for future public health efforts had been planted.

THE FATHER OF EPIDEMIOLOGY

Cholera, caused by the bacteria *Vibrio cholerae,* causes profuse, watery diarrhea. The diarrhea can be so severe that profound dehydration can develop in hours, leading to shock and death. The disease caused severe epidemics throughout history and was typically believed to be due to miasmas — bad air.

In 1844, John Snow (1815–58) received his medical degree from the University of London.[38] Interested in respiration, he conducted many experiments to understand breathing with the ultimate goal of saving babies who were born breathless and blue. Coincidentally, it was this research that gave him the insight that the spread of bad air could not be the cause of cholera.[39]

The workers of the notoriously offensive trades such as tanning and soap making provided evidence that being around noxious fumes was not necessarily deadly. Snow observed that the mortality rate of such workers was no higher than the rates in other industries.[40] If the noxious fumes were as deadly as people thought, then these workers would have had much higher death rates.

Snow was a firm believer of the importance of a vegetarian diet, drinking pure water, and abstaining from alcohol. It was this mindset that may have predisposed him to focus on the problems of the impurities in water as a cause of disease. However, he did not develop his novel theory of cholera transmission until the London outbreak of 1848. From his observations treating cholera victims, Snow noticed that the patients' symptoms appeared to be limited to the gastrointestinal tract and reasoned that the causative agent must be ingested rather than inhaled. Snow concluded that the disease must spread by the fecal-oral route.[41]

In 1854, a cholera outbreak around Broad Street in Golden Square, London, allowed him to test his theory. The outbreak began at the end of August when a woman who lived on Broad Street washed her daughter's diapers in water that she subsequently emptied into a house drain. The drain ran several feet from the well of the Broad Street pump. The baby was ill with diarrhea and died on September 2. During the next 10 days, more than 500 fatal cases of cholera occurred within a 250-yard radius of the Broad Street pump.[42]

Snow suspected that the Broad Street pump was the source of the outbreak. He obtained the names and addresses of the 83 people who died during the first three days of September. When he went to inquire at the houses of the deceased, he found that most had indeed gotten their water from the Broad Street pump. On September 7, he attended a meeting at the local parish and persuaded those gathered to remove the pump handle. They took Snow's advice, and the outbreak subsequently subsided.

A follow-up examination of the pump revealed that the nearby cesspool drain was partially blocked. The examiners concluded that the pump shaft had been contaminated by the cesspool; Snow's conclusions were confirmed, and he went on to study the cholera death rates in all of London.

The two main water suppliers to London were Southwark and Vauxhall Water Company and Lambeth Water Company. The Southwark and Vauxhall Water Company supplied sewage-contaminated water from the Thames river. The Lambeth Water Company had moved its water intake source farther upstream where the water was still clean. Snow, and his colleague, Dr. J.J. Whiting, went to every house in which a cholera death occurred and inquired about the water supply.

They used a map to plot the deaths — the first time that a map was used in such investigations. They found that the mortality rate for houses supplied by the Southwark and Vauxhall Water Company was eight to nine times greater than in houses supplied by the Lambeth Water Company.[43] By conducting a meticulous, scientific investigation of the cause of the cholera epidemic, Snow was able to show that water was, in fact, the actual mode of disease transmission. Since that time, his efforts have served as the basis for epidemiologic investigations.

CROSSING BORDERS: EUROPEAN INFLUENCES ON EARLY AMERICAN PUBLIC HEALTH EFFORTS

Cholera eventually made its way to the United States. In 1832, it killed about 3,000 New Yorkers before spreading to New Orleans, where it killed up to 5,000 people. As with yellow fever in the previous century, thousands fled the cities in fear. Subsequent cholera epidemics helped increase public demand for government action, but without convincing data, persuasive arguments to increase government programs and spending were lacking.

Dr. Edward Jarvis (1803–1884), a prominent physician in Massachusetts, was aware of the European efforts to collect vital statistics for social reform. Jarvis played a major role in the passage of the Massachusetts Registration Act of 1842 that mandated the recording of all births and deaths in the state.[44] The American Medical Association, founded in 1847, worked to enact effective registration laws in other states.

Chadwick's report on the sanitary conditions in Great Britain prompted Dr. John H. Griscom, city inspector of New York City, to recommend that the city provide clean water to the poor, build underground sewers, and establish an effective health department. At the time, many families shared a single privy that would overflow into the streets where manure piles, dead animals, and garbage abounded. Stray dogs, pigs, cows, and horses wandered the streets. Wells were inadequate to meet the population's clean water needs.

Griscom's recommendations faced opposition and led to his dismissal from office; however, his unwavering advocacy efforts eventually motivated others to initiate major sanitary reforms. At about the same time that Griscom was working on his report, Lemuel Shattuck (1793–1859), a former teacher and bookseller, conducted a census survey of Boston and found a shockingly high death rate among mothers and infants. He also found widespread cases of tuberculosis, scarlet fever, diphtheria, and other deadly communicable diseases as well as abysmal living conditions for the poor. Motivated by the British and French efforts in sanitary reforms and by his census findings, Shattuck established a Massachusetts Sanitary Commission with the goal of conducting a sanitary survey of the entire state.[45]

In 1850, Shattuck published one of the most important documents in U.S. public health history, known as the Shattuck Report. The report recommended the establishment of a state board of health, local boards of health in each town, and sanitary surveys in local communities. It also recommended environmental sanitation, communicable disease control, vaccination against smallpox, improved child care, and health education programs. During his lifetime, Shattuck's report had no impact whatsoever, but in the following century, it laid the foundation for all public health organization and practice in the United States.[46]

AWAKENINGS: A LONG-AWAITED BREAKTHROUGH

As noted earlier, beginning in the 17th century, in the hospitals for childbirth that had become common in European cities, patients had suffered from puerperal fever. Even though doctors had developed many theories about its transmission, the spread of the disease had not been controlled. In 1842, an outbreak of puerperal fever occurred in Boston, Massachusetts. A physician, Dr. Whitney of Newton, was conducting an autopsy on one of the victims and accidentally wounded himself. He subsequently died from the disease. Dr. Oliver Wendell Holmes, a staff physician at the Boston Dispensary and a founding member of the Boston Society for Medical Improvement, heard about the deaths and was determined to investigate.

Holmes reviewed the literature, including the earlier British reports, and concluded that physicians pass on the disease by transferring the poisonous fluids they get on their hands after conducting autopsies to their unsuspecting patients. He published a report that recommended that physicians should never attend women in labor if they had conducted postmortem examinations of puerperal fever patients, that physicians attending women with puerperal fever should change every article of clothing and allow at least one day to pass before attending another woman in labor, and that they should relinquish their obstetrical practices for at least a month if they attend two cases of puerperal fever within a short time of each other. His fellow physicians attacked and ridiculed his conclusions and recommendations.[47]

But four years later, Dr. Ignaz Semmelweis, an obstetrician working in a Viennese maternity hospital, reached similar conclusions. Dr. Semmelweis observed that after the Viennese medical school began teaching anatomy with cadavers, the health of the maternity patients worsened.[48] This became clearer after the single maternity clinic was split into two when the number of births became too numerous for one obstetrics professor to supervise them all.[49]

Initially, the male obstetrical and female midwifery students received training in both clinics, but this policy changed in October 1840. According to Semmelweis, when the first clinic began to train only male obstetrical students, the mortality rate from puerperal fever increased and was consistently higher than that in the second clinic. Semmelweis was convinced that airborne causes were not responsible for puerperal fever because the two clinics were adjacent and even shared a common anteroom.

When a colleague died of puerperal fever after being accidentally pricked by a student's knife during an autopsy, Semmelweis realized that the physicians were the ones responsible for transmitting the particles that caused the disease to the women in labor.

He insisted that all students and physicians in the clinic wash their hands with chlorinated lime before examining each patient and recorded the decreasing numbers of puerperal fever deaths as a result of the new policy.

He also noted that harmful particles did not necessarily come only from cadavers.[50]

In 1850, Semmelweis's reappointment was denied, and he left Vienna for Budapest, Hungary. After he left the Viennese hospital, the hand-washing policy that he had implemented ceased, and the rates of puerperal fever began to rise. In 1861, Semmelweis published his findings from his work in maternity clinics in Vienna and Budapest. He used data from a maternity clinic in Dublin, Ireland, as control data, since the obstetricians there did not perform autopsies before entering the maternity wards. He found that after the chlorine hand-washing policies were implemented, the death rates in the Vienna and Budapest clinics dropped to the low levels observed in the Dublin clinic.[51]

Like Holmes years before, Semmelweis was attacked by his peers. However, unlike Holmes, who was able to handle the criticism, Semmelweis fell into a severe depression and mental illness. He was admitted to the Lower-Austrian Mental Home in Vienna and died shortly thereafter.[52]

THE GERM THEORY OF DISEASE

The realization in the late-19th century that many diseases were caused by microscopic organisms revolutionized medicine and public health. For the first time in history, people could devise effective preventive and control strategies against infectious disease epidemics. Drs. Louis Pasteur, Joseph Lister, and Robert Koch were the leaders in developing and applying the germ theory of disease.

Louis Pasteur began his career as a chemist, initially focused on studying the acids found in wine. In 1854, however, the minister of public education appointed him professor of chemistry and dean of science at the newly created Faculty of Lille, where he discovered that microscopic organisms, such as yeasts, played a key role in fermentation. In 1857, he introduced the germ theory of fermentation to the Société des Sciences of Lille.[53]

Pasteur's move from chemistry to microbiology continued in 1865 when he was asked to investigate the cause of the devastation of the silkworm industry, a vital part of the economy in the south of France. After five years of intensive work, he discovered that two different diseases were afflicting the silkworms: pebrine (caused by the microscopic parasite *Nosema bombycis*) and flacherie (caused by infected or contaminated mulberry leaves).[54] These findings provided additional proof of the role of microorganisms in causing disease.

Traditionally, the international medical establishment believed that life could emerge from nonliving organic matter. This spontaneous generation theory emerged after centuries of observing mysteries such as maggots arising from decaying meat and rodents magically appearing in stored grain.

Although a number of physicians and researchers had previously identified microscopic organisms in dead humans and animals, they believed that the microorganisms were the *result* rather than the *cause* of disease.

Pasteur recognized a connection among microorganisms causing disease in silkworms, animals, and humans, but most of the medical establishment was unwilling to relinquish its belief in the spontaneous generation theory. A few notable medical leaders, however, agreed with Pasteur's radical ideas.

In 1864, Joseph Lister, a young surgeon in Glasgow, after reading Pasteur's research, became convinced of the role of microorganisms in causing surgical wound infections. To prevent the spread of infection, he performed surgical procedures using antiseptic techniques. At first, Lister was criticized and ridiculed by his peers, but his methods gradually became accepted. Lister gave much credit to Pasteur for his inspiration.

Robert Koch, a young German physician and researcher, established the field of medical microbiology by proving that anthrax could cause disease in animals and by identifying the tubercle bacillus as the causative agent of tuberculosis. Koch made major breakthroughs in research techniques, such as the use of glass slides and cover slips, fixing and staining bacteria, and growing bacterial cultures on solid media.[55]

In 1882, Koch established criteria for identifying and confirming the microbiological cause of diseases. These postulates, known as Koch's Postulates, required isolating the bacterium, cultivating it in a culture medium, and proving its disease causation effects by infecting animals.[56] By using these postulates, Koch discovered the cause of a number of diseases, including *Vibrio cholerae* as the cause of cholera, *Streptococcus pneumoniae* as the cause of pneumonia, and *Clostridium tetani* as the cause of tetanus. Almost 30 years after the 1854 London cholera epidemic, Koch confirmed John Snow's hypothesis that cholera spread by polluted water.[57]

THE CIVIL WAR AND THE CHANGING FACE OF U.S. PUBLIC HEALTH

Major advances in public health in the United States would not occur until after the Civil War—the last major war fought without knowledge of the germ theory of disease. As a result, more soldiers died from uncontrolled infectious diseases than from direct battlefield injuries.[58]

In 1861, Henry Whitney Bellows, pastor of the First Congregational Church in New York City and a social reformer, persuaded President Abraham Lincoln to create the U.S. Sanitary Commission. Bellows was convinced that the only useful relief effort would be an extensive preventive system based on the British Sanitary Commission's relief efforts during the Crimean War. Florence Nightingale had been in charge of these efforts and with her team of nurses was legendary for reducing the death rates of sick and wounded soldiers solely by implementing strict sanitation reforms.[59]

The U.S. Sanitary Commission selected Frederick Law Olmsted, a brilliant but difficult man, as its executive secretary. Olmsted had directed the expenditure of millions of dollars and the work of 15,000 men in the creation of New York City's Central Park. His work gave him an extensive knowledge of public hygiene and sanitation,[60] but Olmstead faced an uphill battle to improve sanitary conditions in the Union army camps.

Sanitary conditions during the Civil War were horrific. Soldiers relieved themselves a few yards from their tents, with resulting fecal and urine contamination everywhere. In 1863, the rates of diarrhea and dysentery approached 50 percent in General Ulysses S. Grant's army. Vermin were common; men suffered from fleas, lice, and mites. Drinking water was typically contaminated, and army doctors used microbe-laden, bloodstained saws to cut off injured limbs. Pneumonia, malaria, yellow fever, erysipelas (an infection caused by *Streptococcus*), smallpox, influenza, and measles flourished in the camps. Soldiers suffered from malnutrition: the typical soldier's diet included poorly preserved salt pork, stale crackers, and desiccated vegetables that had lost their vitamin C content.[61]

Under Olmstead's leadership, the Sanitary Commission participated in virtually all military medical activities despite initial opposition by Secretary of War Simon Cameron and Surgeon General Clement Alexander Finley. After the Union's disastrous defeat at the battle of Bull Run, Olmstead and his colleagues met with President Lincoln to tell him that the medical department was inefficient and that Cameron and Finley were incompetent. Lincoln refused to make changes.

In response, Olmstead began an intensive advocacy campaign, intending to influence public opinion to improve sanitary conditions by publishing a 96-page report in which he described in great detail the Sanitary Commission's goals, activities, and finances. He gave the report to the press, resulting in praise from prominent newspapers. His goal was widespread military medical reform, and, with time, he achieved notable success.[62]

During the Civil War, the ratio of deaths from infectious diseases compared to deaths from battlefield wounds was two to one. This ratio was better than those in previous wars. For example, the ratio of deaths from disease compared to battle wounds during the Mexican-American War (1846–48) was seven to one and during the Napoleonic Wars, it was eight to one. Thanks to Florence Nightingale's efforts, Great Britain, France, Sardinia, and the Ottoman Empire had a ratio of three to one during the Crimean War.[63]

Although the U.S. Sanitation Commission closed in 1865, the sanitation movement continued.[64] Effective municipal health departments and state boards of health were established. On March 5, 1866, the New York State Legislature approved the creation of the Metropolitan Board of Health, the first permanent health department in the United States. Four years later, the board reorganized as the New York City Department of Health. In 1869, Massachusetts established the first state board of health.[65]

POSTWAR PUBLIC HEALTH DEVELOPMENTS

In its early years, public health in the United States was solely the responsibility of local and state governments. Public health at the national level began in 1798 when John Adams signed "An Act for the Relief of Sick and Disabled Seamen," which provided funds for the medical care of merchant seamen. In 1871, after the Civil War, that program evolved into the Marine Hospital Service and eventually became the Public Health Service.[66]

Dr. John Maynard Woodworth, an 1862 graduate of Rush Medical College in Chicago, distinguished himself as Union General William Tecumseh Sherman's chief medical officer during Sherman's "March to the Sea" and was appointed the supervising surgeon (later, the surgeon general). Woodworth adopted a military model for his medical staff and created a cadre of physicians who could be mobilized and deployed where they were needed and were directed by a central, nonpolitical administration.[67]

In 1872, Dr. Elisha Harris and nine colleagues founded the American Public Health Association (APHA) with the goal of advancing sanitary science and promoting the practical application of public hygiene.[68] Scientific justification for sanitation and hygiene had finally arrived as advances in microbiology, pathology, and chemistry progressed rapidly.

Unfortunately, politics often impeded progress. In the 1880s, New York City's government, including the health department, was accused of widespread corruption and negligence. Experienced public health professionals had been replaced by incompetent political appointees. Increased publicity on the health department's practices eventually led to a major shakeup, new leadership, and reinvigorated effectiveness.[69]

In 1877, a deadly yellow fever epidemic hit New Orleans, spread up the Mississippi River, and focused national attention on quarantine policy. Congress passed the Quarantine Act of 1878, giving the Marine Hospital Service quarantine authority. Woodworth's victory was temporary, however. His arch-rival, Dr. John Shaw Billings, an army expert on hospitals who had wanted Woodworth's job, managed to transfer the quarantine authority to the newly formed but short-lived National Board of Health. Nevertheless, under Woodworth's leadership, the Public Health Service ultimately became the backbone of U.S. federal public health in the 20th century.[70]

In September 1892, ships from Hamburg, Germany, with cholera victims on board, were quarantined in New York harbor. In response to the looming crisis, the New York City Board of Health quickly created the Division of Pathology, Bacteriology, and Disinfection in the Department of Health. Dr. Hermann M. Biggs, a rising star at Bellevue Medical School, was chosen as the director of the division and its new laboratory. The laboratory, the first of its kind in the nation, would apply the new science of bacteriology to solve public health problems.[71]

Biggs had shown an interest in public health early in his career. His medical school thesis was titled, "Sanitary Regulations and the Duty of the State in Regard to Public Hygiene." In 1885, as the director of the Carnegie Laboratory of Bellevue Medical College, Biggs accompanied a group of children who had been bitten by a rabid dog for treatment with the rabies vaccine at Dr. Louis Pasteur's laboratory in Paris, France.[72] Nine years later, as director of the New York City Department of Health laboratory, he sailed to Berlin to learn about the diphtheria antitoxin from Dr. Robert Koch. Briggs subsequently returned to secure funding for similar work in New York City.[73] Under Biggs's leadership, the New York City Department of Health laboratory revolutionized the practice of public health and became a model for other health department laboratories around the world.

THE BEGINNINGS OF INTERNATIONAL HEALTH

Four international sanitary conferences were held, in Paris (1851 and 1859), Constantinople (1866), and Vienna (1874). Issues of concern to the Europeans, such as cholera, dominated the meeting agendas, and the participants from the Americas were disappointed. South Americans were concerned about yellow fever, since a number of epidemics, spreading from Argentina, Brazil, Paraguay, and Uruguay, had killed thousands of people. Participants from the United States were also concerned about yellow fever, particularly after a major outbreak occurred throughout the Mississippi River Valley in 1878 that caused nearly 20,000 deaths.[74]

In early 1881, a fifth international sanitary conference was held in Washington, D.C. Ten diplomats from the Americas, including Carlos J. Finlay, a Cuban physician famous for his work on yellow fever, attended. Finlay announced on February 18, 1881, that the transmission of yellow fever required an insect vector: the mosquito, *Aedes aegypti* (then called *Stegomyia fasciata*). This breakthrough in the understanding of the disease allowed countries to develop control measures against its spread.[75]

Inter-American cooperation began to take hold as a series of Pan American Sanitary Conferences were held generally every four years to promote regional communication and collaboration. The first, held December 2–5,

1902, appointed an organizing committee that included a number of prominent scientists, such as Dr. Finlay of Cuba. This organizing committee recommended that an International Sanitary Bureau (ISB) be established and resolved that in the event of an epidemic, national health authorities would be responsible for disease control efforts in their own countries. The committee agreed to hold meetings in the Americas with officially authorized delegates every two years. The conventions profiled success measures taken by member countries to combat yellow fever.

Five years after the ISB was established in the Americas, a group of European countries set up an Office International d'Hygiene Publique to be headquartered in Paris. The ISB subsequently authorized formal relations with the European organization. Further collaborative efforts were suspended during World War I.[76]

PANDEMIC INFLUENZA IN THE EARLY 20TH CENTURY

At the turn of the 20th century, enormous numbers of immigrants poured into the United States, straining its public health capacity. From 1881 to 1898, 9 million people immigrated to the United States. After 1898, the number of immigrants swelled to include approximately 15 million people over the next 22 years.[77]

The surgeon general and the Public Health Service, rather than the individual states, were responsible for examining the health of all incoming immigrants and for quarantine enforcement. A series of laws beginning in 1891 and the Quarantine Act of 1893 defined this authority. In 1915, approximately 25 medical officers were assigned to screen groups as large as 5,000 people a day. Physicians would systematically and rapidly screen the immigrants as they ascended a flight of stairs for signs of debility or shortness of breath. Immigrants were also examined for various diseases, but less than 1 percent were denied entry to the United States for health reasons.[78]

Dr. Rupert Blue was the surgeon general during the deadly 1918–20 influenza pandemic. He was promoted to this office in 1909 after his predecessor died unexpectedly. Blue was a weak leader who failed to heed warnings and prepare for the crisis. He blocked a funding request by Dr. George McCoy, the director of the Hygienic Laboratory,[79] to do research on pneumonia even though Congress had given his agency authority to study "diseases of man and conditions affecting the propagation thereof."[80]

Blue did nothing to prepare the Public Health Service for the coming pandemic even though he published comments warning about it in the *Memphis Medical Monthly*. Most of the nation's physicians and nurses were overseas caring for the soldiers fighting in World War I, and he neglected to confront that reality. He defended his inaction by minimizing the potential threat of the disease.[81]

Blue also failed to issue orders on what to do about influenza-ridden ships. On June 30, 1918, the British freighter *City of Exeter,* which was docked at Philadelphia with dozens of crewmembers deathly ill from influenza, was released from quarantine.[82] Not until after the disease had spread around the country, killing thousands, did Blue finally ask the U.S. Congress for money. In response, Congress appropriated $1 million for the Public Health Service, but it was too little, too late.

In essence, because of Blue's poor leadership, local communities had to confront the pandemic without any federal help. Leaders in a few small localities took matters into their own hands by implementing stringent protective sequestration policies. They prevented members of their communities from leaving, and they prohibited visitors from entering. Some were able to take advantage of natural geographic barriers and had time to prepare. Most important, they secured the full cooperation of their community members in implementing their policies. The communities that stringently followed them had very few, if any, cases of influenza.[83]

In the end, the 1918–20 influenza pandemic killed somewhere between 50 to 100 million people worldwide.[84] In the United States, almost 700,000 people died, including many young adults.[85] It was one of the largest, deadliest epidemics in recorded history.

The Great Depression in the 1930s fueled debate of the role of federal public health in relation to state and local public health. The tradition of federal public health agencies providing assistance to the states had grown.[86] Dr. Leslie Lumsden, an epidemiologist working out of the Hygienic Laboratory, helped spawn a number of local health departments. For example, after investigating a typhoid fever outbreak in Yakima, Washington, he recommended the formation of a county health department to improve sanitation.[87]

In contrast, Dr. Hugh Cumming (surgeon general from 1920 to 1936) supported federal research activities but opposed federal involvement and support for state and local public health. Lumsden had wanted to be surgeon general, but Cumming got the job, and President Herbert Hoover's administration did little for public health.[88]

THE BEGINNINGS OF THE WORLD
HEALTH ORGANIZATION

The 1920s were a time of accelerated economic growth in the Americas with the expansion of industry and agriculture. Europe was crippled by World War I, so the United States gained increasing prominence in the

Western Hemisphere. Between the two world wars, three international health organizations formed: the International Sanitary Bureau of the Americas, the Office International d'Hygiène Publique (OIHP), and the Health Section of the League of Nations established in 1920 in London.[89] Only the International Sanitary Bureau of the Americas continued as an independent body while the other two organizations eventually became the World Health Organization.

In 1929, the members of the renamed Pan American Sanitary Bureau Directing Council drafted a constitution and statutes which were approved in 1934 at the Ninth Pan American Sanitary Conference. The Great Depression brought a dramatic reversal of the growing South American economies, and health conditions deteriorated. However, World War II did not diminish inter-American cooperation; instead, it brought increased organization and resources as public health workers played an increasing role in the military.[90]

President Franklin D. Roosevelt's New Deal attempted to address public health in the United States. He appointed Dr. Thomas Parran, a commissioned officer in the Public Health Service and former head of the Venereal Disease Division, to be surgeon general. Parran had a broad vision of public health and advocated greater federal involvement in state and local public health. Aided by the Social Security Act of 1935 and Title VI funding, Parran oversaw federal grants to develop state and local comprehensive public health services.[91]

The advent of World War II required that public health services be expanded. The Public Health Service Act of 1944 authorized the commissioning of nurses, sanitarians, scientists, and veterinarians. The U.S. Commissioned Corps (uniformed public health professionals) quadrupled in size and included women and nonphysicians. After the war, the development of the United Nations contributed to an increasing global perspective, with the formation of the Surgeon General's Office of International Health Relations. Parran subsequently played a major role in the formation of the World Health Organization.

World War II's greatest contribution to public health was the establishment in 1942 of the Malaria Control in War Areas (MCWA) program in Atlanta, Georgia. The program involved swamp drainage and the administration of poison that killed insect larvae in an attempt to control malaria throughout the South and the Caribbean. Its mission expanded to include typhus and other tropical diseases that might be found in service personnel returning from overseas duty.

Dr. Joseph Mountain, a protégé of Lumsden and head of the Office of Public Health Methods for the Public Health Service, was determined that the Atlanta program would continue after the war. He envisioned that it would be a major national public health program that would monitor infectious disease outbreaks, educate and support state and local public health agencies, and conduct field research. On July 1, 1946, MCWA became the Communicable Disease Center, the forerunner of the Centers for Disease Control and Prevention. In 1948, Parran was not reappointed surgeon general by President Harry Truman. The Public Health Services' era of extraordinary expansion was over.[92]

At the end of World War II, delegates from 50 nations met in San Francisco to establish the United Nations. Dr. Szeming Sze, a Chinese physician who received his medical training in London, participated in the founding of the World Health Organization and kept a journal of his experiences.[93] Dr. Sze wrote:

> Before the conference opened, the U.S. and U.K. delegations had consulted each other and had agreed that no questions in the field of health would be on the conference agenda. These consultations had not included the Chinese, Brazilian, the Norwegian or any other delegation, so that when Dr. da Paula Souza [a Brazilian representative] and I met with Dr. Karl Evang of the Norwegian delegation for a medical luncheon one day soon after the conference opened, it was perfectly natural, not knowing then about the U.S.-U.K. consultations, that we should agree among the three of us the question of establishing a new international health organization should be put on the conference agenda.[94]

Dr. Sze, as a delegate from China, was able to get the Chinese delegation to initiate the proposal. He drafted a resolution calling for an international health conference of the member states with the goal of establishing an international health organization. This draft resolution was shown to dozens of people in the various delegations to get their support.

The Chinese and Brazilian delegations formally submitted the document. Brazil had been included in order to get support from South America. However, Dr. Hugh S. Cumming, former U.S. surgeon general and director of the Pan American Sanitary Bureau (PASB), strongly opposed the integration of that organization into the new international health organization. In 1947, Dr. Cumming was replaced as PASB director by Dr. Fred Soper, a former Rockefeller Foundation research scientist. Dr. Soper agreed that that PASB would serve as the World Health Organization regional office for the Americas.[95] In 1948, the World Health Organization formally came into existence.

THE HIV/AIDS PANDEMIC

HIV/AIDS is a modern-day plague and a devastating global pandemic that has been decimating populations in Sub-Saharan Africa, Asia, and

Eastern Europe. The virus is believed to have originated from infected African monkeys that people killed and ate.[96] Since viral transmission requires contact with body fluids, such as semen or blood, the virus has not infected the general public, but rather, those individuals who acquired it through sexual contact, sharing of contaminated needles or blood products, occupational injuries, or contaminated organ transplantation.

Unlike smallpox and the other ancient plagues, HIV/AIDS has a prolonged course that can last for decades. There is no vaccine at present, but there are antiviral medications that can keep the infection at bay. Availability of these medications to millions of people in poor countries was limited until June 2001 when a special session of the UN General Assembly met and adopted a resolution declaring a political commitment to addressing the global HIV/AIDS crisis.[97]

Dr. Peter Piot, head of the UN AIDS program from 1996 to 2008, is credited with making political leaders understand the devastating effects of HIV/AIDS on nations' economic, political, and social institutions. He helped increase funding for HIV/AIDS treatment and lower the price of antiretroviral drugs so that millions of infected individuals in poor countries could afford them. During his tenure, funding for the disease rose from about $250 million in 1996 to about $10 billion in 2008.[98]

The virus's impact on history is still unfolding, and politics, as much as the availability of pharmaceuticals and other control measures, appears to be a critical factor in how far the disease will spread.[99] For example, some prominent elected officials in South Africa doubt that AIDS is caused by a virus but is, rather, due to the use of illicit drugs and unhealthy living. Some believe that Western societies are forcing their medications on African nations as a form of exploitation. Controlling this epidemic would be hard under the best circumstances and virtually impossible under a government that doubts the internationally recommended prevention and treatment guidelines.[100]

South Africa has not been the only country in which politics have impeded public health efforts. In the United States, politics also hindered an effective public health response. In 1981, President Ronald Reagan appointed Dr. C. Everett Koop, a distinguished pediatric cardiac surgeon at the University of Pennsylvania and an antiabortion proponent, to be surgeon general.[101] During Reagan's first term in office, he prevented Dr. Koop from addressing the growing AIDS crisis because many conservatives believed that the victims of AIDS, predominantly homosexuals and intravenous drug users, brought the disease upon themselves because of their immoral behavior. In 1983, Edward Brandt, the assistant secretary of health, excluded Koop from the Executive Task Force on AIDS largely for political reasons.

In 1986, almost five years after the AIDS epidemic was first recognized, Reagan asked Dr. Koop to prepare a report on the disease. After meeting with scientists, community activists, AIDS patients, and religious leaders, Dr. Koop carefully wrote a report that treated AIDS not as a moral issue, but as a public health crisis. The report discussed the nature of the disease, transmission risks, and prevention strategies such as condom use and sex education for children.

Dr. Koop was concerned that Reagan's policy advisors would remove crucial public health information, so he distributed report drafts to the Domestic Policy Council (being careful to prevent leaks by retaining all copies of the draft document himself). He then printed 20 million copies to be distributed to the public. On October 22, 1986, he held a press conference to release the report. Conservatives were outraged, but Dr. Koop believed that his report was consistent with his dedication to scientific integrity and Christian compassion. The AIDS epidemic spread unabated until Dr. Koop forced White House officials to treat it as a public health crisis.

PUBLIC HEALTH PAST, PRESENT, AND FUTURE

Before the discovery of the germ theory of disease, societal responses to epidemics were based on a variety of beliefs, some more effective at disease control than others. A few enlightened individuals, such as Holmes, Jenner, Semmelweis, and Snow made significant contributions to public health without understanding the underlying causes of infectious diseases. They, like many other individuals throughout history, met criticism and opposition before there was gradual acceptance of their novel ideas.

The French Revolution radically changed European society and influenced medical leaders to promote the idea that public health should be a government responsibility. Subsequent hygienic movements and influential reports on poverty and disease, particularly the Chadwick and Shattuck reports, contributed to the advancement of public health.

Koch's and Pasteur's germ theory of disease revolutionized societies' understanding of the causes and spread of diseases and provided scientific justification for public health, hygiene, and sanitation policies. Public health advances have dramatically improved life expectancies in the parts of the world where those principles are applied. Unfortunately, many nations, primarily in the developing world, still do not have clean water, food, and air.

The United Nations estimates that by 2050 the human population will reach 9 billion people.[102] Human activities to meet global population demands have already led to environmental degradation, climate change, and the emergence of new diseases. The international public health community has made some efforts to address the rapid spread of emerging and reemerging diseases such as HIV/AIDS, Severe Acute Respiratory Syndrome, and multidrug resistant tuberculosis with new international health regulations and increased disease surveillance efforts.[103]

In some ways, public health has become a victim of its own success. Plagues such as cholera and yellow fever that once randomly devastated wide swaths of societies are rare, or in the case of smallpox, eradicated. However, new disease threats are emerging.[104] Political leaders must be continually persuaded to support public health. Since microbes do not recognize political borders, all nations must work together to ensure global health.

Chapter 3

MICROBES AS WEAPONS

The headquarters of the secret Japanese Biological Warfare program, completed in 1936, was located in Ping Fan, Manchuria. During the years that followed, the Japanese program killed thousands as scientists tested new weapons in their facilities, and untold more died during field tests. They contaminated wells with typhoid, injected unsuspecting people with vaccines spiked with cholera, fed children anthrax-laced chocolates, and dropped plague-infected fleas over open countryside.[1]

BIOWARFARE AND BIOTERRORISM
THROUGH THE AGES

Such deliberate use of infectious diseases to sicken or kill others for political or military gain is not new. Although rarer than the use of conventional weapons, documented cases of biowarfare and bioterrorism have occurred throughout history.

In the sixth century BCE, the Assyrians used ergot of rye, a mycotoxin, to poison the wells of their enemies.[2] Three hundred years later, Hannibal hurled poisonous snakes onto enemy ships during the Battle of the Eurymedon.[3] In the 14th century, Mongols catapulted plague-infected corpses over the walls of the Crimean city of Caffa, hoping to spread the disease among its residents. The citizens of Caffa disposed of the mountains of dead bodies by dumping them into the sea, but they contaminated their own water supply in the process.[4]

During the French and Indian War in 1763, Pontiac, an Ottawa chief, along with allied tribes, besieged Fort Pitt because the British reneged on a number of promises they had made to gain Native American help against the French. During the siege, British Captain Simon Ecuyer, who was in charge of the fort, sent out smallpox-infected blankets and a silk handkerchief to Native Americans outside the fort. Lord Jeffrey Amherst, the British commanding general of the North American forces, supported this tactic in a letter to Colonel Henry Bouquet, who was bringing rein-forcements to Fort Pitt: "You will do well to try to inoculate the Indians by means of blankets, as well as to try every other method that can serve to extirpate this execrable race."[5]

ADVANCES IN THE 20TH CENTURY

It was in the 20th century, however, that bioterrorism and biowarfare became far more technologically advanced and sophisticated. Scientists realized in the 19th century that microscopic organisms caused many dis-eases, revolutionizing medicine and public health. Unfortunately, for every scientific discovery that has saved lives, opportunistic individuals have sought ingenious ways to exploit it for power and wealth—at further cost to human life.

Germany was one of the first nations to have a biowarfare program. The agents of choice were anthrax and glanders, the causes of zoonotic diseases that primarily affect livestock but can also kill humans. During World War I, Germany used germs to sabotage Norwegian, Romanian, Spanish, and U.S. livestock, mainly horses and mules that were used for transportation.[6] German biowarfare was not limited to the battlefield. Sabotage within the United States included bombing munitions depots and infecting livestock.[7]

Anton Dilger, an American-born, German-educated physician, became Germany's key germ saboteur in the United States. He and his brother Carl, a brewer, rented a house in Chevy Chase, Maryland, and built a bio-weapons laboratory in the basement. The Dilger brothers infected guinea pigs with glanders (*Burkholderia mallei*) and anthrax to test the germs' effectiveness as killers. The germs were then injected into horses and mules that were en route to the British Royal Army. Some of their efforts were successful: a number of horses sailing from the United States to En-gland had to be thrown overboard because they were sick with glanders.[8]

Whereas Germany's World War I biological sabotage program targeted animals, a Japanese biological warfare program 15 years later focused on humans. Ironically, the roots of the Japanese program were established in the 1925 Geneva Disarmament Convention that had outlawed chemical and biological warfare after the horrors of World War I. During World War II, Japan developed its massive biological warfare program under the leadership of Major Shirō Ishii.

Ishii, an army physician, was ambitious, patriotic, ingratiatingly persistent, and had well-connected, powerful contacts. He developed his idea for the program after reading a report on the 1925 Geneva Disarmament Convention, written by First Lieutenant Harada, a physician and Japanese War Ministry delegate to the conference.[9] After reading the report, Ishii concluded that if the prospect of biological and chemical warfare created such universal fear, Japan must use it to gain superiority over other nations in future wars.[10]

Ishii also read an article by Dr. Leon Fox, a major in the U.S. Army Medical Corps, in the March 1933 issue of *Military Surgeon* titled "Bacterial Warfare: The Use of Biological Agents in Warfare." In his article, Fox argued that biowarfare was not possible since disseminated microbes could be destroyed by heat, cold, and even sunlight; however, he did concede that anthrax spores and bubonic plague might be militarily useful.[11] Ishii disagreed with Fox's conclusions and embraced the idea of biological warfare with an enthusiasm unmatched by any of his colleagues.

In 1932, Ishii arrived in the occupied city of Harbin, the capital of the Heilongjiang province in northern Manchuria, to set up his program. The Japanese army had given him a large initial sum of 200,000 yen per year[12] from a secret account to build and run his research facilities. He had Chinese laborers begin construction of a large facility outside of the city. Everything was done in secret; the laborers were required to wear eye shields so that they could not have a clear vision of what they were building.[13]

Research in the secret facilities included both animal and human experiments. Human subjects were initially infected with three zoonotic diseases (anthrax, glanders, and plague), but Ishii expanded his research to include poisons, electrocution, and frostbite studies. If the subjects did not die from their ordeals, then they were killed to ensure secrecy. The initial facility in Beiyinhe lasted for five years, after which Ishii had it destroyed to hide the evidence.[14]

From 1936 until Japan's surrender in 1945, Ishii built at least 18 research units in occupied China and additional units in Burma, Singapore, Rangoon, and other sites. This network of facilities was officially and collectively known as the Water Purification Bureau, named after a water purification unit that Ishii created to help counter a cholera epidemic that had killed 6,000 Japanese soldiers, but in actuality, they were research facilities conducting human experiments. Ping Fan, the enormous base of operations for Ishii's network, was located 24 kilometers from Harbin and housed the infamous Unit 731, the site of some of the most horrific experiments.[15]

Like the Nazi physicians who conducted experiments on their death camp prisoners, the Japanese physicians justified their actions in the belief that their human subjects were inferior beings who were being sacrificed for the betterment of the superior races. They told the local Chinese population that the facility was a lumber mill and then referred to their prisoners as *marutas,* meaning "logs."[16] In addition to killing thousands of people, including captured U.S. soldiers, within the research facilities, Ishii and his fellow scientists conducted field experiments on civilian populations. According to some estimates, the use of biological weapons researched in Unit 731 may have resulted in as many as 200,000 deaths in China alone.[17]

Like the German program before it, the Japanese program reached into the United States. In 1939, Naito Ryiochi, a young Japanese physician, tried to acquire the yellow fever virus from the Rockefeller Institute in New York City. His first unsuccessful attempt was followed by a $3,000 bribe to a technician. When that failed, the world famous Japanese bacteriologist Dr. Miyagawa Yonetsugi approached Dr. Wilbur Sawyer, Rockefeller's laboratory director, to get a supply of the virus. Although all efforts failed, they did raise concerns of what the Japanese might be attempting.

Belgium, Canada, France, Great Britain, Holland, Italy, Poland, and other European countries had bioweapons programs even though they were signatories to the 1925 Geneva Protocol. Great Britain conducted field-testing with anthrax spores at Gruinard Island in the north of Scotland. The island remains contaminated with anthrax spores and is closed to the public.[18]

THE ROLE OF THE UNITED STATES

The United States was the last of the major powers to develop a bioweapons program. After Japan carried out several aerial plague attacks in China from 1940 to 1941, Washington became interested in biological warfare.[19]

Compared to the cost of developing nuclear weapons in the Manhattan Project, bioweapons were inexpensive and had the potential to be far more deadly. When World War II ended, U.S. military officials granted Ishii and his colleagues immunity from war crimes in order to gain their cooperation in providing information about their human experiments.

In 1942, President Franklin Roosevelt approved a secret U.S. program to develop bioweapon capability. In August of that year, George W. Merck, president of Merck Company, a pharmaceutical manufacturer, became head of the War Research Service that contracted government agencies and private institutions to begin research on biological warfare.[20] In

April 1943, Detrick Air Field, near Frederick, Maryland, was acquired and commissioned as Camp Detrick and the construction of four biological agent production plants began. In 1944, the biological warfare program was transferred to the War Department and split between two agencies: the Chemical Warfare Service (CWS) and the U.S. army surgeon general. The CWS was responsible for research, production, defense, and foreign intelligence. The surgeon general was to work with the CWS on defense.

Like the Japanese, U.S. scientists focused much of their work on zoonotic diseases such as anthrax, brucellosis, and psittacosis. Brucellosis is a bacterial disease of livestock, and psittacosis is a bacterial disease of birds. Both can spread to humans. Plant killers including rice fungus, 2,4-dichlorophenoxyacetic acid (known as VKA for "vegetable killer acid"), and defoliants were also studied.[21] The United States worked with Great Britain to develop large arsenals of microbes such as anthrax and brucellosis, and, like Great Britain, the United States conducted open-air testing.[22]

In the United States, open-air testing was performed not only over open fields, but over populated metropolitan areas as well. For example, on September 26 and 27, 1950, the U.S. Army sprayed the bacteria *Serratia marcescens,* which was believed to be harmless, from a ship toward San Francisco. Two days later, 11 patients at Stanford University Hospital in San Francisco developed infections from a highly unusual organism: *Serratia marcescens.* One patient died. Because the infection was so uncommon, the physicians caring for these patients published a report on the outbreak, but the episode was forgotten until nearly 30 years later when a reporter uncovered information that the army had used this bacteria for open-air germ warfare tests.[23]

On December 22, 1976, the victim's grandson, a lawyer, read about the tests in the *San Francisco Chronicle* and discovered that his grandfather had died from the bacteria that had been used for testing. He and his family sued the government, but, unfortunately, the judge in the case had a reputation for being biased in favor of the military and the family lost the case. They appealed to the U.S. Court of Appeals, which refused to overturn the decision. A petition for a hearing before the U.S. Supreme Court was denied.

It took a series of three well-publicized mishaps during the 1960s to end the U.S. offensive biological warfare program. Ironically, none of these incidents involved biological weapons, but rather chemical weapons. Over a two-year period from 1966 to 1968, the United States carried out a series of sea dumps of chemical weapons. Termed Operation CHASE for "Cut Holes and Sink 'Em," the military placed surplus mustard and nerve agents, including sarin and VX, into containers and faulty, leaky rocket hulls and sank them in the ocean.[24]

In March 1968, at the Dugway Proving Ground in Utah, nerve agents drifted out of an aerial testing area and onto nearby ranches, killing thousands of sheep. And on July 8, 1969, in Okinawa, Japan, 23 U.S. soldiers and one civilian were accidentally exposed to sarin while cleaning sarin-filled bombs. Fortunately, none of the victims died, but the incident generated concern about the dangers of storing chemical weapons. Each event led to bad publicity for the program, congressional investigations, and public outrage over environmental contamination.[25]

In November 1969, Congress passed Public Law 91–121, banning open-air testing of lethal chemical weapons and imposing controls on testing and transportation of such agents within the United States. At the same time, President Richard Nixon renounced the use of biological weapons, limited research to defensive purposes only, and resubmitted the 1925 Geneva Protocol to the U.S. Senate for ratification. Five years later, nearly 50 years after it was initially proposed, the Senate ratified the protocol and President Gerald Ford signed it into law.

Nixon's actions helped prompt the international community to develop a supplement to the 1925 Geneva Protocol, known as the "Biological Weapons Convention" (BWC). Opened for signature on April 10, 1972, this supplement was the first multilateral disarmament treaty that banned the production and use of an entire category of weapons. The BWC prohibited the development, production, acquisition, transfer, stockpiling, and use of biological and toxin weapons. Great Britain, the Soviet Union, the United States, and other nations signed the BWC treaty in 1972 and ratified it in 1975.[26] Unfortunately, the treaty lacked any formal mechanism to monitor compliance. This weakness led to distrust between nations, illustrated by the Soviet Union, which did not believe that the United States had terminated its biological weapons program.

THE ROLE OF THE SOVIET UNION

Despite signing and ratifying the BWC, the Soviet Union built an enormous biological weapons program. Yury Ovchinnikov, a microbiologist and vice president of the Soviet Academy of Sciences, believed that Russian biology was falling behind that of the West. In 1972, he asked the Ministry of Defense to develop agents for biological warfare. The ministry was not easy to convince, so Ovchinnikov successfully sought support from Soviet leader Leonid Brezhnev. In 1973, Brezhnev issued a secret decree that founded Biopreparat, a massive biowarfare program with thousands of employees and facilities spread throughout the country.[27] The Soviet biowarfare program weaponized pathogens, such as the tularemia and anthrax bacteria and the smallpox and Marburg viruses, among other deadly pathogens.[28] The program was not uncovered until 1989 when one of its top scientists, a microbiologist named Vladimir Pasechnik, defected to the West.[29]

A second Soviet defector, Kanatjan Alibekov (Ken Alibek), spent 17 years as a physician and researcher in Biopreparat. In December 1991, after visiting the former U.S. facilities at Fort Detrick in Maryland, the Dugway Proving Ground in Utah, and the Pine Bluff Arsenal in Arkansas, Alibekov was convinced that the Americans were not conducting offensive biological weapons research.

In 1992, Alibekov quit his position in Biopreparat and was subsequently placed under close surveillance by Russian agents and threatened by officials from the Kazakh Defense Ministry. Alibekov and his family secretly immigrated to the United States, where he spent the next year being debriefed by U.S. officials about the Soviet Union's biowarfare programs.

In April 1992, President Boris Yeltsin signed a decree banning offensive biological weapons research, and in September, Russia, the United Kingdom, and the United States signed an agreement to convert their biological weapons facilities into centers of scientific cooperation and exchanges. Despite these positive developments among nations, events that followed raised concerns about subnational organizations and single individuals committing acts of bioterrorism.

TERRORIST ACTS BY GROUPS AND INDIVIDUALS

In September 1984, the Bhagwan Shree Rajneesh, a cult that had bought a 64,000-acre ranch in Wasco County, Oregon, committed the first large-scale act of bioterrorism in U.S. history.[30] Cult members poisoned local residents with *Salmonella typhimurium* placed in restaurant salad bars. Residents suspected deliberate contamination, because relations between the locals and cult members had deteriorated significantly over land-zoning rules.

Federal and state health officials did not believe that the cult would commit such an act and concluded that there was no evidence for bioterrorism, even though almost 1,000 people developed symptoms and more than 750 had laboratory tests confirming *Salmonella*.[31] One year after the outbreak, the cult leader accused some of his followers of stealing money and using microbes to make people sick; he demanded a government investigation.

Investigators discovered a secret laboratory with a strain of *Salmonella* identical to the one that had caused the outbreak a year before. The commune's germ warfare chief, Ma Anand Puja, was a 38-year-old nurse of Philippine origin who was known by some as "Nurse Mengele." She and a colleague ordered *Salmonella typhimurium* from the American Type

Culture Collection (ATCC) in order to sicken the local townspeople so that they could not vote in the county elections. She and Ma Anand Sheela, the cult leaders' secretary, received 20-year sentences but were released after less than 4 years for good behavior.

In the mid-1990s, a cult in Japan named Aum Shinrikyo also became interested in bioterrorism. Founded in the late 1980s by Shoko Asahara, a partially blind Japanese yoga instructor who sought world power and domination, the cult recruited thousands of followers in many countries, including Japan, Germany, Australia, and the United States. A number of cult followers had been top students and scientists at elite universities and major corporations.[32]

By 1995, Aum Skinrikyo had accumulated more than $1 billion in assets through steep membership fees, a chain of meditation centers, and land holdings.[33] Asahara shrewdly blended science fiction, religion, metaphysics, and modern technology to create an apocalyptic message and vision that appealed to many of the young, talented, and alienated members of society. He preached that the end of the world was imminent and that only cult members would survive. The cult bought buildings in downtown Tokyo and built laboratories. To ensure that the world would end as foretold, three key cult members led efforts to develop weapons of mass destruction.[34]

Hideo Murai, a 30-year-old astrophysicist, was the cult's chief scientist. While working as a physicist at Kobe Steel, he had read one of the cult's books on yoga and extra sensory perception (ESP) and decided to join. He worked on developing a high-energy plasma cannon that would burn off living tissues and a fixed-star reflection cannon that would melt everything in its high-powered beam.

Dr. Ikuo Hayashi, a cardiovascular surgeon, conducted heinous experiments on humans. He gave people drugs, implanted electrodes in their heads, and administered electric shocks to wipe out their memories. The cult's goal was complete mind control. Hayashi ran the cult's clinics and oversaw the torture and murder of a number of followers.[35]

Seiichi Endo had been doing genetic engineering research at Kyoto University's viral research center but quit to become the health and welfare minister for the cult. He cultured bacterial weapons such as anthrax spores and botulinum toxin.[36] Between 1990 and 1995, the cult unsuccessfully tried to release botulinum toxin from a moving vehicle and anthrax spores from the top of a Tokyo office building. It switched to sarin, a deadly nerve agent and, unfortunately, was more successful.

On March 20, 1995, cult members placed packages containing sarin on five different trains in the Tokyo subway system. They punctured the bags with sharp umbrella tips and ran out, leaving the unsuspecting passengers to breathe the deadly vaporous fumes. Almost 3,800 people were injured, 1,000 required hospitalization, and 12 people died.[37] Aum Shinrikyo demonstrated that one group could unleash catastrophe on a city.

Seven years after Aum Shinrikyo used sarin, an unknown assailant(s), possibly a microbiologist at a U.S. army medical research facility, used weaponized anthrax spores in envelopes to kill five people and terrorize thousands.[38]

Such events illustrate that nations are not the only entities capable of carrying out major attacks against societies. Subnational groups and individuals have demonstrated that they are not constrained by moral or ethical values against using weapons of mass destruction to achieve their goals. People who welcome death or have apocalyptic visions are not deterred by the dangers that these weapons pose or by the threat of retaliation.

EMERGING CONCERNS

Rapidly evolving scientific knowledge and technologies are providing the tools to create even more deadly biological weapons than those that already exist. There have been experiments with potentially dangerous results. For example, researchers in Australia bioengineered a mousepox virus in order to infect mice and make them infertile: the ultimate goal was to reduce the mouse burden on the continent. Instead, they inadvertently made the mousepox virus highly lethal and killed 60 percent of the mice in the experiment, even those that had been previously vaccinated.[39] If the results of this experiment were extrapolated to make the smallpox virus (a relative of the mousepox virus) more lethal, then vaccination would not protect the public in the event of a bioterrorist attack. The results would be disastrous.

Other experiments have shown that deadly viruses can be created de novo. Researchers have been able to reconstruct a fully functional and infectious poliovirus using chemically synthesized oligonucleotides, which are genetic building blocks for life. They demonstrated that anyone could theoretically create a dangerous virus from purchased organic chemicals.[40]

To address the growing concerns about the inherent dangers of life sciences research, the National Academy of Sciences released a report in 2004 making recommendations to the scientific, security, and policy communities. The recommendations included educating the scientific community about these dangers, reviewing experiments as to their potential for misuse, creating a national advisory board to advise the federal government, and harmonizing oversight of international research.[41] Some of the report's recommendations, such as the creation of the National Science Advisory Board for Biosecurity (NSABB), have been carried out. The

NSABB released a draft report in April 2007 discussing ways to reduce the risk of life sciences research being used for malevolent purposes.[42]

Bacteria, viruses, fungi, parasites, and other microscopic pathogens are a part of life on earth. Humans cannot conquer them but instead need to learn how to live with them so that they do not cause deadly epidemics. Throughout history, individuals have struggled to understand how epidemics began and spread. Some have devised treatment and containment strategies, but it was not until Pasteur, Koch, and their colleagues developed the germ theory of disease that epidemic control efforts started becoming successful. Unfortunately, the germ theory of disease has also equipped individuals with the ability to spread death and terror. The dangers of naturally occurring and deliberately set epidemics will not disappear: the challenge is to have leaders who can prepare for and confront them when they arise.

Chapter 4

RISING TO THE OCCASION

POLITICAL LEADERSHIP DURING INFECTIOUS DISEASE CRISES

Political leadership is absolutely critical during an infectious disease crisis. How political leaders handle these crises can determine the ultimate success or failure of their administrations. Although these leaders typically defer to local fire and police chiefs in appropriate situations, severe public health crises necessitate active political participation. Political leaders who defer to their public health bureaucrats, if such people exist, often still find themselves at the center of decision making as the crisis worsens.

The political leaders most intimately involved with infectious disease epidemics or bioterrorist attacks would arguably be those at the local level because these events typically begin at local facilities, hospital emergency rooms, or physicians' offices. Leadership problems can develop as the severity of the crisis escalates: some elected officials rise to the occasion, but others do not. Successful political leaders develop good working relationships with public health and medical experts *before* crises develop. They consider public health expertise as a strategic asset in government and learn their own roles and responsibilities if a public health disaster develops. Successful political leaders develop what if scenarios, identify resources, and establish game plans.

Marcus, Dorn, and Henderson have written about the concept of *meta-leaders*—individuals who make decisions beyond their official lines of authority in order to facilitate collaboration across agencies and jurisdictions.

This concept is an effort to overcome traditional silo thinking that characterizes many political and bureaucratic leaders.[1] The challenge with relying on meta-leaders to emerge during crises is that individuals must be willing to act beyond their official job descriptions, potentially risking disciplinary actions if their decisions or actions are subsequently deemed inappropriate.

One could argue that elected officials are natural meta leaders. They have the ultimate authority and are in a position to facilitate cross-organizational and cross-jurisdictional collaborations. In the United Kingdom, senior ministers (elected officials) meet daily to facilitate cross-government communication and collaboration during crises. The senior ministers' roles are clear: they provide high-level coordination while the leaders of agencies carry out the operational aspects of crisis response.[2]

The following three case studies, two in the United States and one in Canada, illustrate how three different mayors handled their leadership roles during infectious disease crises. In the first two crises, the mayors essentially served as meta leaders. They made critical decisions and facilitated cross-organizational efforts.

In the first case, Mayor Glen Gilmore of Hamilton Township, New Jersey, established relationships and identified resources before the crisis developed. Despite not having a public health leader at the local level, his relationship with a local private hospital administrator made a tremendous difference in saving lives. In the second example, Mayor John Norquist of Milwaukee, Wisconsin, had initially deferred decision making to his public health commissioner. Nevertheless, disputes between the health commissioner and the water works superintendent required him to make a critical public health decision. In the third crisis, Mayor Mel Lastman of Toronto, Ontario, Canada, failed to provide effective political leadership, and the deputy mayor had to assume control.

ANTHRAX ATTACK, FALL 2001, HAMILTON TOWNSHIP, NEW JERSEY

Tuesday, September 18, 2001, was a warm, clear day in New Jersey. Sometime during that day, near the heart of Princeton Borough, someone placed envelopes contaminated with deadly anthrax spores in a mailbox. The letters were addressed to news media companies and were transported 10 miles away to a large postal sorting and distribution center in Hamilton Township. Covering more than 280,000 square feet, this facility processed 2 million pieces of mail a day.[3] En route to their final destinations, the letters passed through the facility's high-speed sorting machines that inadvertently aerosolized the spores out of the envelopes.

At the end of September, Robert Stevens, a 63-year-old photo editor at a supermarket tabloid in Florida, began to feel ill with fever, malaise, and muscle aches. A few days later, he awoke confused and vomiting. His wife took him to a nearby medical center where Dr. Larry Bush, an infectious disease specialist, treated him. Stevens received a diagnostic workup and a spinal tap. His spinal fluid appeared cloudy, signaling an infection. The medical center's laboratory performed the initial tests on the infected spinal fluid, and the Florida Department of Health laboratory provided the confirmatory results. Dr. Bush had identified the nation's first case of inhalational anthrax due to bioterrorism.[4] Stevens died on October 5.

About the same time that Stevens became ill, Teresa Heller, a 45-year-old mail carrier in New Jersey, noticed a red sore near her wrist. It itched and after a few days, blistered and turned into a brown scab.[5] By the time she saw her doctor, the scab had gotten larger and turned black, and her wrist had started to swell. Her personal physician did not know what it was and referred her to an orthopedist. The orthopedist could not help her either and sent her to a plastic surgeon. The plastic surgeon hospitalized her and scraped out the blackened, dead tissue from her wrist.

Heller's doctors identified her condition after a case of cutaneous anthrax was publicly reported in New York City. Her doctors sent a sample of the wrist scrapings to the New Jersey Department of Health and Senior Services (NJDHSS) for initial testing, and ultimately to the Centers for Disease Control and Prevention (CDC) for confirmatory testing. The CDC did not respond to the plastic surgeon's request to see the laboratory report, forcing the doctor to learn on television that the specimen tested positive for anthrax.[6] Heller became the first person in New Jersey identified to have anthrax.

The announcement of Heller's condition came after anthrax-laced letters addressed to government officials were mailed and delivered to the same postal facility in Hamilton Township.[7] Drs. George T. DiFerdinando Jr., the acting commissioner of health, and Eddy Bresnitz, the state epidemiologist for the NJDHSS, made the difficult decision to close the Hamilton Postal Facility on October 18, without the support of the CDC or the U.S. Postal Service.[8] Neither the CDC nor the U.S. Postal Service believed that the state had any proof that the facility should close, but the doctors held firm. In addition, they initiated an intensive statewide search for more victims. The search found three additional confirmed cases and one suspected case of cutaneous anthrax, and two more infected with inhalational anthrax.[9] The two individuals with the deadly inhalational form of anthrax worked alongside each other and right next to the high-speed machines that sorted the contaminated letters.

During the statewide investigation, the NJDHSS laboratory was inundated with thousands of specimens to test for anthrax. Environmental samples gathered at the postal facility demonstrated that the entire facility was contaminated, vindicating the doctors' decision to close it down.[10] Before these results were available, Dr. DiFerdinando recommended, again without CDC approval, that all 1,000 federal postal employees who worked in the Hamilton facility should be treated with prophylactic antibiotics.[11] Because the CDC disagreed with this decision, it refused New Jersey access to the national pharmaceutical stockpile.[12]

Dr. DiFerdinando had no choice but to recommend that the postal workers see their private physicians because there was no public health infrastructure in the county that could meet the workers' needs. On a Friday night, he went on television and urged the postal workers to see their own doctors. Unfortunately, many of these physicians were unavailable during the weekend, and workers who did manage to get prescriptions were unable to have them filled because pharmacies had run out of the antibiotics.

Mercer County, where the attacks took place, includes New Jersey's state capital, Trenton. Situated in the middle of the state, the region is densely populated with more than 350,000 people[13] and includes Princeton University and several major pharmaceutical companies. At the time, Mercer County did not have a county health department. This meant that during the anthrax crisis, there was no one in charge locally and there were no facilities or personnel in place to treat the postal workers.

To fill the public health leadership void, Hamilton Township Mayor Glen D. Gilmore sought help from Christy Stephenson, the chief administrator of Robert Wood Johnson University Hospital in Hamilton.[14] She ordered 18,000 antibiotic pills; the mayor sent a police car to South Jersey to pick up the supply and deliver it directly to the hospital. Over the next three days, the private hospital served as the de facto county health department and treated the postal workers. Fortunately, no one died in New Jersey, but the anthrax-contaminated letters initiated a chain of events that killed five, sickened seventeen, and terrorized thousands.

MAYOR GLEN D. GILMORE, HAMILTON TOWNSHIP, NEW JERSEY

Glen D. Gilmore was elected mayor of Hamilton Township, New Jersey, in November 1999. He was born in the small blue-collar town of Manville, New Jersey, and was the first in his family to graduate from college. He showed an early interest in public service by becoming a legislative aide, at age 16, to a New Jersey assemblyman. Gilmore trained at the U.S. Army Airborne School at Fort Benning, Georgia, and was honored with the title of "Distinguished Military Graduate" for displaying outstanding leadership qualities, academic achievement, and high moral character. He was later awarded the U.S. Army Commendation Medal for "exceptionally meritorious service."[15]

Mayor Gilmore had the foresight to establish an Emergency Task Force after September 11, 2001, to anticipate a future crisis. He even identified, in advance, a place to acquire antibiotics if they were needed. This case illustrates that elected officials who serve communities with weak or nonexistent public health leaders will likely have to fill the role of the bureaucratic leader.

Because state and local public health capabilities were lacking, Mayor Gilmore was forced to serve as both political and public health leader. He improvised a public health response with the local private hospital to provide antibiotics to the exposed postal workers and arranged to have a police car collect the antibiotics. Without the presence of an extraordinary leader like Mayor Gilmore, who was willing to take charge, the absence of a public health leader may have led to unacceptable consequences for the public health and welfare of the community.

The following is an account of the crisis in Mayor Gilmore's own words.

> As mayor of a community, I consider public safety my number one priority. I will do everything in my power to keep it safe, and I will not wait for the county, state, or federal government to act. There are over 90,000 people in Hamilton Township; September 11, 2001, changed our world instantly.
>
> I developed an Emergency Task Force after the terrorist attacks of September 11. The task force's charge was to deal with emergency preparedness, hospitals, and schools. While the concept seemed far-fetched, bioterrorism was part of the charge as well. At the first meeting, I asked the hospital representative, Christy Stephenson, to identify a supplier for Ciprofloxacin [Cipro, the antibiotic to treat anthrax].
>
> I first heard about anthrax in Hamilton Township from a retired state trooper who works with me. He had just heard on the news that the Trenton post office had been identified as the site from where the four anthrax letters had been mailed. He had a hunch that it was the Hamilton post office and not the Trenton post office.
>
> I turned my car around and headed to the Hamilton postal facility. The place was swarming with U.S. postal inspectors, FBI, and CDC. No one bothered to notify local law enforcement.
>
> I showed my mayor's badge and was given a briefing. Federal officials had identified the facility as the place of origin of the anthrax letters that had killed several people. I asked the feds, "Who's at risk?" They answered, "No one." They went on to say that the only person who was at risk was the

person who opened the envelope at the end of the mail stream. I then asked, "Who's going to decide for possible building contamination?" The scene then became like a Fellini film. The FBI said that the building should be tested, but they were only there for the criminal investigation. They said that the CDC or state health officials would decide. Then they began pointing fingers at each other as to who would decide the full extent of testing inside the expansive post office building.

It was clear to me from the beginning that no one had a sense of who was in charge. I felt that there was a general unwillingness to take charge and risk making a mistake—by everyone. I learned in the military that "when in charge, take charge." The governor called and [said] that I should report to his office immediately.[16] He told me that people at the postal facility were exposed, and possibly infected, to the anthrax spores. That began the debate as to whether or not to close the facility. I was waiting for the folks from the state to say so. I said, "Of course you have to close it."

Over 1,000 federal postal workers work at the facility. I thought the U.S. president should be in charge. Not a blip. The feds never asked what we were doing, and they didn't do anything to provide antibiotics for their workers.

The next day, I went to the postal facility cafeteria and began to talk to the workers. They told me that they use air blowers on the conveyor line to keep dust off, and they were concerned. It was demonstrated that dirt could blow out of envelopes. They were afraid they were exposed to anthrax.

I went to see Christy [Stephenson] at the hospital. I told her about the possible contamination of the postal facility. I asked her to go and get a stockpile of Cipro with an open credit for the mayor. I knew enough that anthrax was deadly and needed to be rapidly treated. I sent a police car to get the supplies.

At first I was told by a state health official that there wasn't any risk. Then later, the state health department issued a recommendation that everyone who had worked in the facility would have to get Cipro. You're talking over 1,000 workers.

I asked, "How are we going to arrange for that?" I was told that they should see their personal physician to get their prescription. Pharmacies were running dry and there was a shortage. I told the state that I had a large supply of Cipro already and could mobilize my health department and set up a clinic at the local hospital. The state health official told me that he couldn't recommend any particular hospital. I thought he had the worst mind-set.

What is the priority and primary responsibility of government? We need to cut through red tape and recommend a way to save lives. The mayor is entrusted with public health. Christy didn't have any hesitation or express any concern about exposing the hospital to liabilities—the only concern she expressed was about public health.

I told the press that the postal workers were at risk and that starting the next day we would have a free clinic to provide the antibiotics. The post office notified no one to come to the clinic. The post master of the Hamilton facility claimed that he hadn't been able to notify anyone at that point because the names and contact numbers of the workers were in the sealed facility. I thought that was nonsense and just an excuse. There was more concern about the equipment in the facility than there was for the people who worked there. Shame on the federal government for not stepping forward and caring for their own employees.

We kept the clinic at the hospital open around the clock. Our [municipal] public health facility was not adequate in size. The hospital had a better facility and supplies. The press got the word out and the next day 300 people came. There was definitely a vacuum in leadership, and I had to step up to the plate. The federal government did an abysmal job with a lack of leadership at the top. The president of the United States is the person ultimately in charge. He could look to the governor and mayor for assistance, but he is the one most able to muster every resource needed. I figured our efforts during the anthrax attacks would be a stop-gap until the feds came in, but this didn't happen.[17]

CRYPTOSPORIDIUM OUTBREAK, SPRING 1993, MILWAUKEE, WISCONSIN

Lake Michigan supplies the drinking water for the 800,000 residents of the city and surrounding municipalities of Milwaukee, Wisconsin. On March 11, 1993, chemists at the South Side water plant in Milwaukee faced repeated problems with the water treatment process. The chemists were struggling with a new chemical, and, to make matters worse, the plant's filtration system began to falter.

A little more than a week later, on March 21, the level of turbidity in the water from the water plant increased to unprecedented levels.[18] Milwaukee residents began calling Milwaukee Water Works (MWW) officials with complaints about foul-smelling brownish water. Many of the people who called were given a variety of explanations for why the water was dirty, cloudy, and smelly. MMW employees and the Milwaukee Health Department assured them that the water was safe to drink.[19]

Officials at the MWW did not contact the health department about the water problems or about the telephone complaints.[20] According to hospital records, between April 4 and April 6, the number of people complaining of severe watery diarrhea, cramps, and vomiting was well above normal levels.[21]

On April 5, the health department began receiving calls from the public about the outbreak. The department began an investigation into the crisis and received anecdotal reports that emergency rooms in the area were filling up. Local pharmacies called with reports that antidiarrheal medicines were selling quickly. City health officials suspected that a gastrointestinal virus was spreading because bacterial tests in the hospital laboratories were negative.[22]

The city health commissioner, Paul Nannis, called the state health department and the CDC to help investigate the outbreak. But it was not until Dr. Thomas A. Taft, an infectious disease specialist, called the health department in the late afternoon on April 7 to report that his patient at West Allis Memorial Hospital had tested positive for cryptosporidium, a waterborne parasite, that the health department began to recognize the cause of the outbreak.[23] People panicked as they sought bottled water. Emergency rooms were inundated with calls asking for guidance, but the city health commissioner and the MWW superintendent, Jesse Cooks, could not agree on a plan.[24] In the end, the mayor made the decision to advise Milwaukee residents to boil their water.[25]

Accusations abounded. City officials blamed animal waste from dairy farms for contaminating the rivers that feed Lake Michigan.[26] Mayor Norquist wanted to impose fines on farms that contaminated the waterways.[27] The medical chief of the health department, Dr. Thomas Schlenker, blamed the water officials for acting evasively and lying; although he later apologized.[28] Wisconsin State Senator Charles Chvala (D-Madison) blamed Republican Governor Tommy Thompson for weakening a pollution control bill the previous year.[29]

The mayor was credited for taking action: advising citizens to boil water, shutting down the offending water treatment plant, and holding daily press conferences. His performance was given high ratings by Milwaukee residents in a newspaper poll, even though they were generally distrustful and cynical toward the city government.[30]

The outbreak was estimated to have sickened more than 400,000 people, hospitalized 4,400 people, and killed more than 100.[31] It was the largest documented waterborne outbreak in U.S. history.[32]

MAYOR JOHN NORQUIST, MILWAUKEE, WISCONSIN

John Norquist was elected mayor of Milwaukee, Wisconsin, in 1988 and served until 2004. He was born in Princeton, New Jersey, and was the second of six children. Norquist showed an early interest in politics by joining a teenage Republican club briefly while still in high school, and he became a registered Democrat in college. He marched in antiwar protests in 1968 and 1969.[33]

At the age of 24, Norquist ran for the state legislature in Wisconsin and won; he quickly developed a reputation for being intelligent and hard working. He decided to run for the legislature because he opposed a freeway project that the incumbent supported. His victory ensured that the Stadium South Freeway was never built.[34]

Mayor Norquist first found out about the outbreak from Paul Nannis, head of the health department:

> They had noticed a pattern of flu-like symptoms breaking out in the Milwaukee water service area. It had been going on for a number of days. The health department suspected cryptosporidium. The water department doubted that the Milwaukee water could be the source.
>
> The health department had invited a number of people to a meeting, including the state epidemiologist, Dr. Jeff Davis. The health department and the water department were in disagreement. The water department leadership team seemed to want to avoid blame. Commissioner Nannis wouldn't have been comfortable getting into a big public fight with the water department. Paul needed the elected executive to step in and sort things out.
>
> At the meeting, there was a glass of water on the table. I turned to Jeff [the state epidemiologist] and motioned towards the water. I asked him, "Would you drink that water?" He said, "No." I said, "Well, if you won't drink the water, then no one else should either." I then arranged to go on TV and radio and order people to boil their water. The head of the water department seemed miffed when I took sides with the health department. He realized later that he had no reason to be angry when it was proven that the water was the source of the illness.
>
> I think the role of elected officials is to be out front. It is easier for bureaucracies to work together if the elected leader leads. If elected leaders don't take the lead, then bureaucracies have a harder time working together. In a major crisis, elected officials can help to facilitate information sharing and coordination of efforts among the media, bureaucracies, and the public.
>
> I decided not to hide in my office. But you have to be careful to not appear to be showboating. I made sure that as soon as something was learned, I'd share it with the press and public. People with immune system problems were of a special concern. They were [at] high risk from the contaminated water. I think it is important to share information with the public as soon as possible. You have to make sure information is accurate and not let rumors build up.[35]

SEVERE ACUTE RESPIRATORY SYNDROME (SARS), SPRING 2003, TORONTO, CANADA

Outbreaks of atypical pneumonia began appearing in China's Guandong Province in the middle of November 2002, but no clinical samples were collected from these earliest cases. It was not until December 17 that a chef who regularly had contact with the exotic animals used in Chinese cuisine became one of the first identified cases of Severe Acute Respiratory Syndrome (SARS). The chef infected his wife, two sisters, and seven health care workers.[36]

It was not long before similar cases began cropping up in the vicinity. Between December 26 and January 20, 28 cases developed in the nearby city of Zhongshan. On January 31, a 46-year-old male seafood merchant was admitted to the Second Affiliated Hospital of Zhongshan University. He infected more than 30 hospital staff members before he was transferred to another hospital, where he infected 20 more medical staff. During the same time, 19 of his relatives became ill.[37]

China failed to notify the World Health Organization (WHO) about the spreading disease until three months after the outbreak began,[38] when China's Ministry of Health announced 305 cases of atypical pneumonia in Guangdong Province, with one-third of those cases being health care workers. International health officials expressed frustration that China had not sought their assistance and refused their offers of aid.[39]

Shortly after the initial outbreak, the disease began crossing country borders. In mid-February, one physician from the Second Affiliated Hospital in Guangzhou traveled to Hong Kong and became a major source of the SARS outbreak in that city and beyond.[40] The doctor stayed at the Metropole Hotel, where he inadvertently infected other hotel guests, who spread the disease around the world to Canada, Ireland, Singapore, the United States, and Vietnam.[41] Health officials in Hong Kong speculated that many, perhaps all, of the people he infected spent a few fateful minutes with him while they waited for an elevator at the Metropole Hotel.[42] By mid-March, 300 more cases were reported outside of China.[43]

One of the hardest hit cities outside of China was Toronto, Canada. Toronto is Canada's largest city and the capital of the province of Ontario. All of its 2.5 million residents, served by 19 acute care hospitals, are insured for all essential health services through a universal, provincial insurance plan.

Landing at Toronto's Pearson International Airport on February 23, Suichu Kwan, a 78-year-old Toronto woman, and her husband were returning from their 10-day trip to Hong Kong, where they had stayed at the same Metropole Hotel as the infected doctor.[44] In the days following her return, Mrs. Kwan became feverish with flu-like symptoms and died from SARS at her home on March 5, but not before infecting several family members, including her 44-year-old son, Chi Kwai Tse, who died on March 13.[45] That night Tse's wife, five-month-old baby, and sister became ill and were rushed to the hospital. A man in his 70s, who had been in the hospital bed next to Tse, also became ill and was moved to intensive care.[46]

Dr. Sandy Finkelstein, Tse's physician at the Scarborough Grace Hospital, called Dr. Barbara Yaffe, the associate medical officer of health and director of communicable disease control at the Toronto public health agency, to tell her that he thought he had a tuberculosis outbreak on his hands. He also called his colleague Dr. Allison McGeer, a microbiologist at Mount Sinai Hospital, to warn her of the possible outbreak. By the time Tse died, the public health agency had already begun an investigation.[47] The agency reported Toronto's first case of SARS on March 13, only one day after the World Health Organization issued its first global alert about atypical pneumonia. Scientific teams around the globe rushed to identify the infectious agent.[48] It was initially believed to be a paramyxovirus, which can infect humans and animals and commonly causes respiratory infections with flu-like symptoms.[49]

On March 21, scientists from the National Microbiology Laboratory in Winnipeg announced that they had isolated a metapneumovirus, previously known to cause only mild respiratory infections, from sampled Canadian patients.[50] Scientists from the CDC suspected that a coronavirus was the cause of SARS.[51] University of Hong Kong microbiologists stated that SARS was definitely caused by a new strain of coronavirus that was similar to a strain found in cattle.[52] Crown-like in appearance, coronaviruses commonly cause colds in humans but can cause severe disease in animals.

As new cases were being reported and deaths began to mount, Ontario's commissioner of public health, Dr. Colin D'Cunha, commented in a press release and conference that

> Unless someone has been in direct contact with individuals who have the disease, the probability of getting infected is slim, near zero.[53]

The Scarborough Grace Hospital emergency room temporarily closed its doors to all new patients in an attempt to contain the outbreak. Mount Sinai Hospital had four isolation rooms for SARS patients.[54] Toronto Public Health set up a hotline for people to call if they had questions or concerns about SARS.

By March 27, Dr. Sheela Basrur, the Toronto medical officer of health, announced that people who had set foot in the Scarborough Grace Hospital on March 16 or later would have to place themselves under quarantine for 10 days from the time of the visit. This policy had the potential to affect thousands of individuals. The Ontario premier, Ernie Eves, declared a provincial emergency. D'Cunha announced that isolation beds were going to be opened in different locations in the Toronto area. Dr. James Young, the Ontario commissioner of public safety, said that the general risk of contracting SARS was small and they didn't want to cause unnecessary panic in the community.[55] When there are too many spokespersons or leaders, the public can receive conflicting information.

The Red Cross refused to help provide food to the quarantined families because too little was known about the illness and how it was spread. The David Lewis Public School in Scarborough was temporarily closed after three kindergarten students were sent home with fevers.[56] A special clinic at the Women's College Hospital was set up to screen patients suspected of having SARS. Canadians were urged not to travel to China, Singapore, or Hanoi. Traces of the SARS coronavirus, from samples taken from the SARS victims, were found in the federal Canadian laboratory in Winnipeg.[57]

WHO asked Canadian officials to screen airline passengers to halt the spread of SARS. Passengers would be asked if they had any symptoms such as fever, coughing, or breathing troubles, and whether they could have possibly been exposed to someone with SARS. The federal Health Minister Anne McLellan said that the government was "seriously considering" WHO's request even though there were a number of practical problems in its implementation.[58]

A doctor and nurse who returned from a 16-day tourist trip to China complained that the screening efforts at Toronto's Pearson International Airport were inadequate. Instead of having nursing staff on hand, an immigration officer merely asked the doctor if he had "any symptoms" of SARS. The doctor, Dr. Marshall Redhill, was also disappointed by his inability to get through to the Health Canada hotline, which was jammed with calls.[59]

On April 23, WHO issued a travel advisory for Toronto. Speaking publicly for the first time since SARS hit Toronto, Mayor Mel Lastman condemned WHO for advising against nonessential travel to Toronto.

He said, "I've never been so angry in my life. I want them here tomorrow. I think they are doing this city and country a disservice. What I am doing is sending a message to this CDC group, whoever the hell they are." He was corrected that it was not CDC, but rather WHO, that had issued the advisory.[60]

On the night of Thursday, April 23, in the wake of the advisory, Mayor Lastman appeared on CNN to allay the fears of those traveling to Toronto. During his interview with *Newsnight* host Aaron Brown, Lastman said,

> They [WHO] don't know what they're talking about. I don't know who this group is. I've never heard of them before. They're located somewhere in Geneva. And they haven't talked to us all. They read the papers and sometimes

the papers exaggerate. They [WHO] want to wait three weeks. In the meantime, they're hurting Toronto badly.[61]

WHO responded to Lastman's complaints by saying that the death of a Toronto-based nursing assistant in her hometown in the Philippines was one of the main reasons for its travel advisory for Toronto. WHO also expressed concerns about three additional possible SARS cases that Toronto may have exported to Australia and to the United States.[62]

In response to the WHO explanation for the travel advisory decision, senior Canadian health officials accused the agency of relying on bad science and being illogical. Dr. Donald Low, the microbiologist in chief at Mount Sinai Hospital in Toronto said, "Even if this [Filipina] patient develops SARS, what has this to do with a travel advisory to a city? Does that mean somebody from California, [who] has SARS, gets on a plane and comes to Toronto and gets sick, is there a travel advisory on California?"[63] His primary complaint was that there had not been a single new SARS case in a week and no community spread in 19 days. If WHO had issued its travel advisory when SARS cases were on the rise in the city, then he would have accepted the decision. He believed that WHO was guided by political concerns rather than facts.[64]

After the WHO travel advisory, the mayor and city councilors united in urging local residents to go about their normal routines and to go out to eat and shop. Lastman announced a $25 million tourism marketing campaign that included $10 million from the province of Ontario, $10 million from the federal government, and $5 million from the city of Toronto.[65]

On May 10, Basur claimed that, "for all intents and purposes, from my standpoint the outbreak is over. It's only a formality to actually declare the emergency itself over for administrative reasons."[66] On May 14, WHO took Toronto off its list of places affected by SARS. It had lifted its travel advisory against the city, which was in effect for six days, three weeks earlier.[67] According to D'Cunha, only 10 people remained in hospitals as probable SARS cases.[68]

After the recovery, the city tried to revive its image by planning a free Rolling Stones concert, but the recovery did not last long. On May 22, Toronto public health officials announced four new suspected SARS cases—two in critical condition—and issued a broad quarantine. They would be the first suspected cases in more than a month. Public health officials insisted that these cases were not infected in the community, but rather through travel or through exposure in a health care setting.[69]

By this time, Toronto health officials, convinced that the SARS outbreak was over, had dismantled their containment team and departed to give lectures on how they had contained the disease. James Young, the

Ontario commissioner of public security, and other medical experts had flown to Hong Kong, Taipei, and Beijing to share their Toronto SARS experience.[70]

By May 26, officials identified eight additional SARS cases and 26 with suspected SARS.[71] Low, the chief microbiologist at the Toronto Mount Sinai Hospital, was the first to admit that something was amiss. During a radio interview, he said, "There's a lot more patients out there that have SARS than we're letting the rest of the world believe."[72]

Health Canada, the Canadian federal government's agency in charge of human health, defined suspect cases of SARS as people who had close contact with a patient with SARS, a fever of 38°C or higher, and a new onset cough or shortness of breath. Suspect cases were reclassified as probable cases if chest X-ray or autopsy findings showed pneumonia and/or severe acute respiratory distress syndrome (also known as ARDS). In the later stages of the epidemic, a blood test became available to test for the associated coronavirus—although it was not 100 percent accurate.[73]

In contrast, the WHO definition of a probable case of SARS was less stringent than Health Canada's. WHO required only that chest X-rays showed evidence of the disease or that a patient's blood test was positive for the coronavirus.[74] The result was that Canada was undercounting its probable SARS cases because some cases did not meet all of its criteria.

Ontario's nurses had had enough. The initial outbreak, which lasted from February 23 to April 21, had been prematurely declared over. The second outbreak lasted from April 22 to July 1, 2003. Nurses were exhausted, and many were underpaid for their efforts. Many were isolated in quarantine. Some quit. And some became critically ill with SARS.[75]

The nurses demanded an independent review to discover why nurses' warnings of a second outbreak went unheeded. Doris Ginspun, the executive director of the Registered Nurses Association of Ontario said, "Nurses [were] giving warning signs—and they [weren't] listened to. We can't continue to allow nurses to ring the alarm bell and not be taken seriously." The nurses tried to tell doctors that there had been more SARS patients, but they were ignored.[76]

In the end, Toronto had 225 people with SARS, of whom 38 died. The vast majority of the people who came down with SARS caught the disease while in a hospital setting. More than 23,000 people were identified as requiring quarantine, but only 13,000 of them complied. The Toronto Public Health hotline received more than 300,000 phone calls.[77]

In June 2003, the Ontario government established an independent commission to investigate the SARS outbreak in Toronto. Justice Archie Campbell, a judge of the Ontario Superior Court of Justice, was appointed commissioner. The commission held six days of public hearings and conducted more than 600 interviews with people connected with the SARS outbreak. The final report was released to the public on January 9, 2007.[78] None of the final recommendations addressed the political leadership during the crisis.

The Toronto newspapers criticized the political leaders, particularly Mayor Mel Lastman, for poor leadership during the SARS outbreak. According to newspaper and television interviews, Lastman knew very little, if anything, about the SARS crisis prior to the WHO travel advisory for Toronto. After the travel advisory, he demonstrated how uninformed he was and actually made statements that worsened the situation. His political leadership had a negative impact on the response, and he was quickly relegated to a secondary role.

Prior to the outbreak, Lastman had been a popular and outspoken mayor, but his performance during the SARS crisis tarnished his reputation. Deputy Mayor Case Ootes filled in because of Lastman's poor leadership. The political leadership focused on the image of the city as a safe place to visit rather than on the outbreak itself. Toronto was fortunate in that the bureaucratic leadership, composed of public health professionals, was competent and capable enough to handle the crisis independently, except for declaring the crisis over before it actually was. But despite the public health professionals' leadership, the media wanted to see and hear from the elected officials.

In a *Globe and Mail* column, Margaret Wente wrote about the mayor's failings:

> What's wrong with Mel? . . . First he decided there wasn't any crisis. Then he went on CNN, wondered who was WHO, got all his SARS facts wrong. . . . A mayor is ultimately measured by how well he reflects the values and self-image of the people he represents. By that measure, Mel is a catastrophe.[79]

An editorial, also from the *Globe and Mail,* summed up the political leadership at all the levels of government during the SARS crisis by stating,

> . . . from the beginning of the SARS outbreak in Toronto, leadership has been astonishingly lacking at all three levels of government. In fact, Prime Minister Jean Chretien, Ontario Premier Ernie Eves and Toronto Mayor Mel Lastman were all vacationing outside the country for various periods as . . . health officials scrambled to corral the spreading disease. Politicians need to be seen and heard often in crises.[80]

DEPUTY MAYOR CASE OOTES, TORONTO, CANADA

Case Ootes first entered municipal politics in 1988 as an East York Councilor.[81] At that time, the municipal government of Toronto was composed of six area municipalities, as well as the regional level of government.[82] As a result of provincial legislation, the six municipalities and regional government merged on January 1, 1998, to form the new City of Toronto. Mr. Ootes was appointed as the first deputy mayor of the newly amalgamated city; he held this position for six years. Here is how he described the crisis:

> Toronto has 2.5 million people, and greater Toronto has over 5 million people. The city's role in the outbreak was to communicate to the world at large that as long as people stay away from hospitals, they would be okay. The outbreak was mainly within the hospital system. Our job was to assure people that Toronto was still a safe city to come to. The city continued to function. Our concern as a city government was the image of the city as a place to avoid. We had to reassure everyone that the city was safe. The mayor had difficulty with interviews—primarily with the American media. He was relegated to a secondary role. After that, I did practically all the interviews with the foreign media. It became a job of public safety. The public felt confident in the professional response, but not in the political response. Elected officials are expected to provide reassurance. The public understands that.
>
> In a crisis like SARS, [you] need to create an image of public confidence—an image of a team. Assure [them] that the political leadership is working with the bureaucracy. You need to have the professional staff around you when giving a daily briefing.
>
> The political leader should be front and center to appear in charge. The public expects this. Individual politicians sometimes fail to understand this. I think the overall response to the outbreak went quite well. The medical response was about as good as it can get. There were quarantine questions. Overall, the public was reasonably happy, but don't give credit to the political leadership.[83]

CONCLUSION

These examples illustrate the critical role of political leadership during an epidemic or bioterrorist attack. In the first example, Mayor Gilmore served as both political and public health leader because of the lack of a public health leader at the local level. He did not have the option to delegate authority and was solely responsible for decisions at the local level. He was the meta leader. He was fortunate that he had a knowledgeable and supportive private hospital administrator to provide the necessary medical support.

Mayor Gilmore stated that he expected more leadership from the federal level. State and local officials who assume that the federal government will come to the rescue will be sadly disappointed. In the United States, public health is a state and local responsibility. In addition, U.S. public health and medical care do not interface seamlessly, which further complicates response capabilities.[84] One could argue that the federal government should have provided health care for the federal postal workers, but there was no medical infrastructure in place to do this: it had to be improvised by the mayor and the hospital administrator.

The public health bureaucracy in Milwaukee, Wisconsin, was mired in a conflict with the water works department. The public health leader and the water works leader disagreed about what to do. Mayor Norquist played a key role by stepping in to resolve the dispute and issuing a "boil water" advisory. Political leaders need to recognize that sometimes they must resolve conflicts between bureaucratic leaders.

Toronto, Canada, had a competent public health bureaucracy that had the support of its elected officials, who delegated decision-making authority to the public health professionals and provided political support. However, the media faulted their poor political leadership since they deferred most of the public communication to the public health professionals. Although journalists want scientific information from the professionals, they want the political leaders to announce their support for the decisions their appointees make. They also want the political leaders to demonstrate that they are on top of what is happening.

In all three examples, the elected officials interviewed found themselves filling leadership vacuums. Mayor Gilmore had to serve as both the political and public health leader and had to improvise a response during the anthrax crisis. Mayor Norquist had to mediate a dispute between two bureaucratic leaders: the public health commissioner and the water works superintendent. Norquist ultimately became the main spokesperson during the cryptosporidium outbreak. Deputy Mayor Ootes stepped in to cover for Mayor Lastman's poor leadership performance.

Chapter 5

SUCCESS FAVORS THE PREPARED PUBLIC HEALTH LEADER

Public health leadership is as important as political leadership during a disease crisis. Public health leaders must work within their public health systems, however robust or weak they may be. In addition, they must communicate and collaborate with leaders from different agencies, jurisdictions, and disciplines.

Problems can arise when public health leaders' expectations or assumptions about their roles and responsibilities, particularly in relation to those of the political leaders, are incorrect. For example, if a public health leader decides that a population needs prophylactic antibiotics after a possible exposure to a deadly agent and announces the decision publicly, he or she could face difficulties if the elected official does not provide political support. This scenario happened in New Jersey during the 2001 anthrax crisis and is described in one of the interviews in this chapter.

To examine the relationships among politics, public health, and medicine, the public health and medical leaders involved in the crises described in chapter 4 were interviewed and asked to discuss their experiences and observations.

ANTHRAX ATTACKS IN NEW JERSEY, FLORIDA, MARYLAND, AND NEW YORK

The examples of crisis response in these four states illustrate the importance of an understood chain of command, an effective local public health infrastructure, and political support during a bioterrorist attack. State and local authorities are responsible for public health in the United States; the federal government primarily provides financial and technical support.[1] Much of the variability in state and local leadership capabilities rests on relationships, competence, and trust.

The following interviews bring out several important points. First, public health leaders who have preexisting relationships with medical leaders in the community have an advantage in receiving early warnings of possible outbreaks. After all, clinicians are the eyes and ears of public health. Public health leaders who work in well-integrated and robust public health and medical infrastructures can handle disease crises even if political leadership is weak.

Second, the relationships between political and public health leaders appear to follow two models: the Giuliani Model, in which the political leader makes decisions with the public health leader's expert advice, or the Glendening Model, in which the public health leader makes decisions with the political leader's explicit support. Problems can develop if there is a misunderstanding between the two leaders as to how their relationship will function. Finally, leadership confusion can arise if responsibility is split between leaders.

New Jersey

Dr. Daksh Patel was a private medical practitioner in Trenton, New Jersey, during the anthrax attack in 2001. Dr. Patel operated independently to treat anthrax victims without any assistance from the local, state, or federal authorities. This is his experience:

> [A woman] came into my office with a simple cough and fever. I thought she had a simple bronchitis and put her on Ciprofloxacin, an antibiotic. She got very sick over the next 24 hours and went to the emergency room. She had fluid in her lungs. We extracted fluid and sent it out for cultures. I didn't know she had anthrax. I thought she had a case of simple pneumonia and put her on broad spectrum antibiotics.
>
> We had no suspicion of anthrax in Trenton. We only found out about anthrax after the cases in New York and Washington, D.C. We also found out about another woman in Cherry Hill [New Jersey] who was also a postal worker. Both got sick as the news broke.
>
> Most of our information came from the federal government. People from the U.S. Army came down to interview us. I never contacted anybody, and the state health department never contacted me.[2]

Christy Stephenson was the president and CEO of the Robert Wood Johnson University Hospital in Hamilton, New Jersey, at the time of the anthrax attack. Her story provides an example of how private individuals and political leaders can work together in times of crisis based on preexisting personal relationships, even in the absence of local public health leadership.

[The Robert Wood Johnson Hospital] focused on the municipality and county. At the state level, [George] DiFerdinando and [Eddy] Bresnitz were the conduit with the CDC [Centers for Disease Control and Prevention]. The Department of Health focused on the state, and Glen Gilmore [mayor of Hamilton], the hospital and town. It had to be coordinated. Because [Glen and I] were on a first-name basis, we acted as one unit, and the community benefited.

We couldn't get antibiotics from the CDC. We went to our supplier and asked if they would procure the antibiotics at the hospital's expense. They came through, and we got the antibiotics in a few hours. DiFerdinando had initially heard that 10 days of treatment would be effective. Later that was extended to 30 days, so the postal workers needed more drugs. The hospital pharmacy director worked with our suppliers to get the medications quickly. Mayor Gilmore sent a courier to pick up the medications from the suppliers.[3]

Dr. George T. DiFerdinando, Jr. was acting commissioner of the New Jersey Department of Health and Senior Services during the anthrax crisis. Without a productive working relationship with the acting governor, Donald DiFrancesco, he was left to make many of the response decisions without the benefit of political support, and he paid the consequences:

I was in charge at the state level. Donald DiFrancesco was the acting governor.[4] He let me lead. When we had our first press conference, the FBI, postal inspectors, and our own state police all wanted to do their own thing. The governor and I shared the podium. He made some statements, and I made a statement. It was a challenge because this was at the end of the administration. People had started moving on, and they were glad to let me do what I wanted to do. They deferred to me medically. They didn't provide, and I didn't ask for, political cover.

There are certain decisions that are good to publicly share with the boss. It is important to have him say, "That's my decision, too." I wasn't sophisticated enough to understand the differences between being liberated to make policy decisions on my own versus having policy decisions shared. I got into a match with the mayor of Hamilton over certain specific issues that I should have shared with the governor's office and passed on for cover so I could keep doing my job.

There were multiple decisions with complex dynamics. The mayor [of Hamilton] and I had differences over using nasal swabs [to test the postal workers]. We had decided to treat people anyway, so it was pointless to take nasal swabs. I couldn't be convinced that the emotional aspect of the workers was worth swamping the [state] laboratory with specimens. That decision affected the rest of our relationship.

I could have used state power to just announce that I would send everyone to the hospital for antibiotics. It would have been good if I had had the governor's support.

After the decision was made by the hospital and mayor [to dispense antibiotics], he was still upset with me. I became his "opponent," and I was doing "bad" things.

The CDC didn't send [its] primary team [to New Jersey] because [it was] distracted with Florida, then New York City, then Washington, D.C. [It was] stretched very thin. [It] sent a reasonable, but not high-ranking, group. [It] said no to the use of [its] antibiotic stockpile, which was a big problem for me. The leader of the CDC team was adamant when we decided to recommend prophylactic antibiotics to the postal workers. Atlanta said no.

The CDC team [members] didn't come to the press conference. I should have walked into the governor's office and demanded that they talk to the senators. I didn't have access to antibiotics. That meant that people had to go to their own doctors. None of us was sure enough to take on the CDC. I should have said that I'm right and they're wrong. I didn't have political backup.

A lot of my difficulty came from a lack of decision-making authority by the CDC team [members]. They had the authority to say no. They made a decision that the anthrax did not aerosolize and that there was no need to close buildings. They gave no input to close the Hamilton postal facility. They neither advised [stopping] it from being closed nor [keeping] it closed.

We had 4 cutaneous and 2 inhalational cases of anthrax.[5] The cutaneous cases appeared to have occurred from a distance from the infected letter. Eddy Bresnitz, the New Jersey State epidemiologist, had talked to people in Florida. They had data that anthrax had spread in their postal facility. That information was not shared, and it would have helped our decisions. We have a lot of politics here in New Jersey. New Jersey stays under the radar. The upside is you get to make your own decisions, but it is also a downside.[6]

Florida

Dr. Larry Bush, a private infectious disease specialist practicing in Palm Beach, Florida, at the time of the attack, diagnosed the first anthrax victim. Through his close working relationship with the director of the local health department, he was able to alert the local public health authorities who had the political support of the local elected official and the resources to coordinate the response.

I've known Dr. Jean Malecki, the director of the Palm Beach County Health Department, for a long time. We had previously worked together on a hospital infection control committee and on county committees.

When I suspected my patient had anthrax, I knew to call Jean because she was in charge here at the local level. The chairperson of the infection control committee is in charge of all infections within a hospital. The infection control coordinator, usually a nurse or lab person, is the first person physicians at a hospital should contact if they have an unusual case. Then infection control decides what to do next. All hospitals have a chair of infection control but not all are infectious disease specialists.

If it is decided that the case is serious enough to call the local or state health department, then the chair of the committee might do that. [The chair] might even call the CDC straightaway if [he or she doesn't] know whom to contact at the local or state level.

Once the disease was diagnosed as anthrax, a large group of people, including local and state health, the FBI, CDC, and law enforcement, showed up at the hospital.

I was stunned when Tommy Thompson, secretary of the U.S. Department of Health and Human Services (HHS), said that Bob Stevens, the first diagnosed victim, had naturally acquired anthrax. I called Steve Wiersma, the state epidemiologist, at the State Health Department and asked him how he let that information get out. There was a lot of misinformation.

The CDC had written an article about anthrax in JAMA [*Journal of the American Medical Association*] in 1999 that said that inhalational anthrax should be considered bioterrorism until proven otherwise.[7] Scientists wrote this paper. The people who were in charge of the anthrax response didn't read the article.[8]

Dr. Jean Marie Malecki was the director of Florida's Palm Beach County Health Department at the time of the anthrax attack.

I was once on the same hospital staff as Dr. Larry Bush. He is a peer [whom] I have worked closely with over the years and have much respect for as an infectious disease doctor. He had a case that was presenting as meningitis but called me with his suspicion of the anthrax bacillus. As we waited for confirmation, I immediately began the epidemiological investigation to be ready if the lab confirmed this suspicion. Soon the meningitis was ruled out, and the confirmation of anthrax arrived.

I led the local investigation for the State of Florida Department of Health and Palm Beach County Health Department. My political liaison, at the time, was Warren Newell, chairman of the Palm Beach County Commission. Newell and all local elected officials were very supportive of our efforts.

After we isolated the source of the anthrax as being in the AMI Building, we immediately closed the facility in the interest of public health. It was then that it became politically charged as many wanted the FBI to take control as a criminal investigation. I felt that it was important that the local persons remain an integral part of the communication strategy and not lose control of the communities' needs. Washington, D.C. and the state took over communication. I was removed from the front lines of TV and print communication, which left people wanting to know what was going on in their local communities. They were left searching for a local credible official.

The public health professionals should be doing the communications as long as they are appropriately trained and competent. Physicians carry credible weight with the public. Politicians should at least have physicians beside them whenever the community's health is at stake.

Our operation is 24/7. We have an on-call line with 14 hospitals, and we have regular meetings with infectious disease physicians. Communication is ongoing.

In Florida, 25 percent of the 67 county health departments are run by physicians. But only three, including myself, are trained in preventive medicine and public health.[9]

Maryland

Dr. Georges Benjamin was secretary of the Maryland Department of Health and Mental Hygiene during the anthrax attack. Politically astute, Benjamin kept his boss, Governor Parris Glendening, in the loop. He recognized that there are always political elements to crises, and he discussed the political challenges he faced when making decisions. His close relationship with the governor helped him gain the political support he needed during the crisis. The governor was happy to let the expert lead and to provide political support when necessary.

I was the state health secretary of Maryland during the anthrax crisis of 2001. The actual event occurred in the District of Columbia, but the index case was a Maryland resident who was exposed in Washington, D.C., and went to a hospital in Virginia. It wasn't clear if it was due to inhalational anthrax. It was not known at the time how he got sick, but he was a postal worker.

We eventually learned that he had carried mail from Brentwood to a facility outside of the Baltimore/Washington International Airport. This knowledge helped focus the investigation on the Brentwood facility. Occupational Safety and Health Administration investigators found anthrax spores all over the Brentwood facility, where high-speed presses, used to process the mail, were found to have spewed the spores all over the facility.

During the investigation, there was concern about contaminated mail from federal facilities directly downstream from the Brentwood facility and from private people and organizations. I got a call from a Maryland banker who told me that he had a postal unit in his bank with similar machines. He wanted to know if his folks were at risk.

We needed to be proactive. I was put in charge of the response for Maryland by the governor. The governor also partially activated the emergency command center, which included the state police, the Department of Environmental Protection, the governor's communication office, and our own communication office.

We sent messages to the media. We offered environmental screening of mail rooms for any business that wanted it and provided broad surveillance to ensure there were no cases in the rest of the community. Our environmental team went in to investigate, but none were positive for spores. Everyone seemed focused on Washington, D.C., not on the areas outside of D.C., despite the real concerns by people in the region. It took awhile to get people to focus on this, even though the health officers of Maryland, Washington, D.C., and Virginia all communicated with one another to coordinate our activities.

A number of issues came up. First, we agreed that we should stop doing nasal swabs since they weren't helpful for deciding on therapy, but people thought that they should have them because they had been done in the Senate Hart building and in Florida. Second, we changed antibiotics from Ciprofloxacin to Doxycycline. Both are equally effective against anthrax, but Cipro is more expensive and harder on the stomach. Unfortunately, the reasons for the change were not communicated effectively. People got the impression that they were treated differently from those in the Senate Hart building. Some people thought they were being given the different antibiotic because of a racial difference between the two groups. We spent a significant amount of time trying to defuse the situation.

Parris Glendening was the governor of Maryland. I reported to him once or twice a day. I made sure to keep him in the loop. I made the programmatic decisions and made sure that I got political support. I think it worked pretty well.

There were a lot of white powder runs that set off a lot of panic. Emergency Medical Services [EMS] was constantly receiving calls. They were responding to events 10, 15, 20, 30 times per day, all around the state. This was happening around the nation, too. Labs were testing powders on mailboxes and counters. Spilled Sweet 'N Low® got picked up and tested. We needed to develop protocols for dealing with this. We worked with police, fire, and EMS to make reasonable decisions regarding anthrax exposure. Usually people just needed to be reassured that it wasn't anthrax.

There is always a political element to crises. At the end of the day, the political official is responsible. If you have a riot, you let the police official make decisions and handle it. It's the same thing with public health. It must be a partnership built on trust. You have to know when to go to them [political officials] for support. It's important to keep them in the loop.

The challenge with some crises is that they might start out as a public health emergency, but at some point, they can go beyond public health and authority is transferred from one person to another. The political leader would have to be involved because [he or she] would be ultimately responsible. The Giuliani model was effective. He had experts to support him. Governor Glendening's approach was also a model.

Of course, it very much depends upon the skills, expertise, and knowledge of the individuals involved. A lot of health departments are run by lawyers or human services directors who may or may not have medical or public health knowledge. Having medical knowledge is absolutely important. Of course, I'm biased because I'm a physician, but in a local health department, the most knowledgeable person is usually the one people trust.[10]

New York City

Dr. Neal L. Cohen was the New York City commissioner of health and mental hygiene in 2001. Cohen explained his role as advisor to Mayor Rudolf Giuliani, who actively led the response to the anthrax crisis.

In order to understand the city's response to the anthrax attacks, it has to be put in the context of the terrorist attacks on September 11, 2001. Mayor Rudolph Giuliani established great credibility with the public during the 9/11 attacks. He was an excellent communicator during that crisis, and the city was still in the crisis mode when anthrax hit. His credibility and relationship to the public were critical in enabling us to gain the cooperation of those impacted by the anthrax letters.

Mayor Giuliani had assembled a Weapons of Mass Destruction [WMD] advisory group during his first term in office with my predecessor, Dr. Peggy Hamburg.[11] During my tenure, he held several tabletop exercises involving bioterrorism led by his Office of Emergency Management located at 7 World Trade Center. The building collapsed on the afternoon of the 9/11 attacks.

In fact, the WMD advisory group was meeting on October 5 at a command center set up at Pier 92 overlooking the Hudson River when HHS Secretary Tommy Thompson announced the confirmed case of inhalation anthrax in Florida. We were meeting to consider bioterrorism as a possible component to 9/11.

One week after the Florida confirmation, we had confirmation from a CDC laboratory that a New York City NBC worker had cutaneous anthrax. I got the call very early in the morning and immediately called the mayor and arranged to meet with him.

When the mayor and I met, we called the CDC director, Jeff Koplan. Koplan said, "The findings were consistent with anthrax." Giuliani shot back, "Is it or isn't it?" Koplan responded, "It is."

Mayor Giuliani scheduled a press conference for later that day. His approach was to get information out to the public as soon as possible. New York City is a media capital. It is important to head off any rumors. We needed to be as direct and candid with the public as possible.

I accompanied Mayor Giuliani to the press conference. He gave an overview of what had happened, and I was called upon to give more detailed information on the public health aspects of the crisis.

The city was very anxious. It had white powder phobia. The labs were overwhelmed with specimens for testing. We used regional labs, including the national lab at Wadsworth in Albany, the CDC, and the U.S. Army Medical Research Institute for Infectious Diseases to help keep up.

The anthrax crisis required both criminal and public health investigations. The mayor pulled both components of the investigation together. He made sure that all of the agencies involved were working effectively together. We also had regular meetings with the CDC. Dr. Steve Ostroff[12] of the CDC National Center for Infectious Diseases was in New York City frequently. He had previously been a regular consultant to New York City on West Nile virus issues. He was helpful and knowledgeable and gained the confidence of the mayor. Our assistant commissioner for infectious diseases, Dr. Marci Layton, was an enormous resource both locally and nationally. Her public health advisories were shared with public health authorities throughout the crisis.

Steve and I gave our advice to the mayor, and he was consistently supportive of our recommendations. We proposed that the city establish a clinic at each media site that had received anthrax letters. We interviewed the workers and established our epidemiological investigation. We needed to know how the letters were handled, who was at greatest risk for exposure, and who would most need antibiotic prophylaxis. We also did nasal swabbing for the epidemiological investigation.

We had hundreds of people at the NBC site who wanted antibiotic prophylaxis, but as the days progressed, fewer people were clamoring for it. We had mental health counselors working side by side with the other health care workers. With each new confirmed case, Mayor Giuliani went with the police commissioner and me to meet with the staff to describe the nature of our investigations. He was very hands on, and it was a very effective way for us to merge both the criminal and public health investigations.

For me, it worked well. I benefited from his experience in responding to media questions. But there is no one-size-fits-all approach. It has to be a team effort with a public official who respects a public health expert's knowledge base and recommendations.[13]

CRYPTOSPORIDIUM IN MILWAUKEE, WISCONSIN

The response to the cryptosporidium epidemic was problematic at the governmental level. The water department denied that the problem was its fault, and the health department deferred the decision to boil water to the political leader. Acting on the advice of local experts, the mayor made the decision to issue a boil water advisory.

Dr. Thomas Taft played a key role in identifying the cause of the 1993 outbreak of the waterborne parasite *cryptosporidium* in Wisconsin. He contacted the director of the city laboratory with his findings.

The epidemic had been going on for about one to two weeks. The people at West Allis[14] had yellow tap water. They called the Water Works and were told that there had been a change in technique, but even so, people didn't want to drink it. We never served yellow water in the hospital. Only certain areas were getting yellow water.

West Allis [Memorial] Hospital was the first hospital hit. An inordinate number of people were sick with diarrhea. The medical staff was sick as well and sometimes had to use the patient facilities when the public restrooms were occupied. Since all [bacterial] cultures were negative, it was thought that [the disease] was viral until a colon biopsy on one otherwise healthy individual showed *cryptosporidium. Cryptosporidium* was usually an organism that infected only the severely immunocompromised. We knew something else was occurring—most likely a waterborne infection. I called Steve Gradus, the director of the city laboratories, about the biopsy result. It turned out to be a citywide problem.

I then contacted Sandy Schroederus at the hospital lab. I wanted to see what was going on with the other specimens. She went back and looked at all the stool specimens. All tested positive for *cryptosporidium.* After that, we knew what was causing people to get sick.

I called Steve back and told him what we found. Steve told Paul Nannis [the city health commissioner]. Paul told the mayor, and the mayor told the city. The mayor issued the recommendation to stop drinking the water. At the time, it was a big step. No other city had made this recommendation before.[15]

Paul Nannis, trained in social work, was the commissioner of health of Milwaukee, Wisconsin, during the *cryptosporidium* outbreak:

[John] Norquist was elected mayor of Milwaukee in April 1988 and asked me to come with him as his city health commissioner. We in turn hired Dr. Tom Schlenker, a physician, who had a strong background in public health. During the outbreak, this team approach worked as we hoped it would.

By Monday, April 5, we knew something significant was happening. We were mapping out cases from community labs, hospitals, medical clinics, and nursing homes. The concentration of the outbreak seemed at first to center on the South Side water plant. There had been a burst of illnesses that had been emerging over the weekend prior to April 5.

On Wednesday afternoon, for a variety of reasons, we believed that the vector was, in fact, water. Some parasite had infected the water. Dr. Tom Taft, a local infectious disease physician, reported to us that he had identified several positive cryptosporidium stool specimens. Just at the same time, Dr. Steve Gradus, our lab director and microbiologist, had done so in our city health department lab. This rare and unusual event was in fact proof that *cryptosporidium* was the agent.

That evening, we gathered a team, including Dr. Jeff Davis [state epidemiologist]; staff from the water department; and Drs. Gradus, Schlenker, and others to meet with the mayor and his staff. There was an initial disagreement as to who should manage the media aspect of the crisis. Jeff Fleming, the mayor's communications director, said that it couldn't be the water department because at the time it had little credibility. He argued that the mayor shouldn't take charge because it might be viewed by the public as a political response. The obvious choice and clear decision was that this was a health issue. The health department would take the lead on it. The health commissioner would be the point person for the crisis.

Once the health department examined the turbidity logs, in retrospect it was clear that a public health scientist should have always been working with the water department in monitoring turbidity. The turbidity levels had spiked significantly but never exceeded federal thresholds. To the water department, not having exceeded these thresholds meant that this wasn't a problem. But from a public health perspective, it obviously was.

At the meeting that evening, the mayor asked Jeff Davis if he would drink the [city's tap] water. When Dr. Davis said no, the mayor decided to issue an advisory to the public to boil water until we were certain that the water was clear of the parasite.

As point person, I did all the national morning talk shows. I never made anything up. It was important to me to never give any information out that we couldn't defend. And we didn't. It helped to earn the respect and trust of the media by not lying to them.

People were dying. Almost all of them were HIV/AIDS patients. The lines between public health and politics had been crossed. Of course the active AIDS community was angry, scared, and frustrated. They wanted answers. We didn't have them when they wanted them. Some local AIDS activists threw vials of blood at the mayor's steps.

What dominates? Politics? Science? The decisions affect many. We got a lot of flak from folks who wanted answers right away. People wanted to know when the boil water advisory would stop. The answer was that until the scientific evidence proved otherwise, we didn't know. The political answer would be to make something up to appease people.

We kept the boil water advisory for eight days, in part because there were few labs that could test the water for cyst or *cryptosporidium*. We needed time to repeatedly test the water until we could assure the public that it was clean. We all wanted this to be an evidence-based, science-driven, healthcare process. Even today, there are those in the water department who refuse to believe, in spite of all the evidence and all the time that's passed, that it was their water that was the problem.[16]

SARS IN TORONTO, CANADA

In Canada, the medical and public health infrastructures are closely integrated. Canada has 10 provinces and 3 territories. Public health is largely organized at the provincial level with health units distributed throughout the country. This is analogous to the U.S. model, which has state-level oversight of local-level public health providers, but the roles and responsibilities of the elected and appointed officials appear to be clearer in Canada than in the United States, where they seem primarily driven by the personalities of the individuals involved.

During the SARS crisis, government ministers provided political support and resources to the appointed officials who made the response decisions. In essence, they followed the Glendening model of leadership, with experts in charge supported by politicians.

Politics was a major issue during the SARS crisis, compounded by political and economic pressures from the World Health Organization (WHO) travel advisory. Despite the challenges they faced, Canadian public health leaders responded to the SARS outbreak about as well as they could have, given the scientific uncertainties that they faced. Their medical and public health infrastructures were integrated and robust enough to handle the stresses imposed by the crisis.

Dr. Donald Low was microbiologist-in-chief of the Department of Microbiology at Mount Sinai Hospital, Toronto, when Sui-chu Kwan and her husband landed in Toronto, bringing SARS to the unsuspecting city:

> One of the problems with the SARS response was that there was dual responsibility between James Young, the Ontario commissioner of public security, and Colin d'Cunha, the Ontario commissioner of public health. They gave conflicting views and opinions and created a huge problem. D'Cunha reported to Tony Clement, who was the minister of health—the elected official "in charge." Young, a coroner, was in charge of disasters such as bombings, and he reported to the minister of community safety and correctional services. In other words, they were equally in charge, but reporting to different ministers.
>
> The province of Ontario has 37 different health units, and each unit is headed by a different medical officer of health. Some might be more draconian than others in their responses. Toronto was more lenient. People were concerned about their own turf. The elected officials were usually in a supportive role.
>
> We run a pretty active community-based research group at the Mount Sinai hospital. We often get asked for advice regarding community-related infections. The index case, a woman, died at her home on February 23. Her son was admitted to Scarborough Grace Hospital on March 7 with a community-acquired pneumonia. He sat in the emergency room 12 to 18 hours before getting admitted to the ICU. He died March 12. There were rumors that he had avian influenza. WHO had announced a new disease.
>
> We began an investigation around March 12 to 14. Our infectious disease person, Allison McGeer, talked to the family members. Several of the family members were admitted to our hospital with what appeared to be this new disease. It was a well-defined outbreak.

Information from Hong Kong on March 15 to 16 through ProMED included a description of seven cases with clinical symptoms of this new disease.[17] The new disease got a name: Severe Acute Respiratory Syndrome or SARS.

By Monday, we were intimately involved. I was asked to join a public health press conference to give the clinical perspective since Allison was off on March break with her family. That week, we had a couple of press conferences. That's how I got involved.

By the next weekend, things were growing. SARS was becoming more of an issue. We were experiencing a much bigger outbreak than we had expected. Around March 16, we recognized that the disease had spread outside of the index family. It was no longer a curiosity. The physician who had first seen the index family got sick. Someone who had been in the emergency room with the primary case [the sick son] was now sick. And it spread to others. We gathered as much information as possible. Health care workers were getting sick.

On March 23, we opened up a wing of a closed hospital to admit health care workers with SARS. It was still not declared a public health emergency. There was no leadership.

Two weeks into the outbreak, on March 26, government officials finally recognized that we had a crisis. We met that evening in the coroner's office to devise a strategy to contain it.

On the 27th, we wrote directives that we sent to hospitals on how to contain the spread. On the weekend of the 29th, we were phoning colleagues across Canada to get them to come and help us write policy. We had no policy. In addition to writing provincial policies, we each had our own hospitals to manage. We were closing our out-patient clinics, restricting access, screening all persons allowed into the hospitals, and canceling services.

Media interest was growing. Iraq was being invaded, so there was little U.S. interest. I think the media did a pretty good job. This was a new disease that was spreading and killing people. They did a good job because we didn't see people panicking. We didn't see people wearing masks on the streets or leaving town.

The most effective strategy was to use the media to get the message out. There was a decision to do a daily press conference, but there should have been one spokesperson. I think the media, however, wanted to hear from more than one person; they wanted to hear other stories.[18]

Dr. Bonnie Henry was the associate medical officer of health at Toronto Public Health during the 2003 SARS outbreak:

I was in charge of emergency preparedness and part of the communicable disease program for Toronto Public Health [TPH].

TPH was notified on Sunday, March 9, about a young man who was admitted to hospital with a concern of tuberculosis [TB]. The TB nurses initiated a follow-up with the family. Over the next few days, we realized that other family members were ill. This was before the WHO and China information became available.

We were aware of a family that had left Hong Kong for a visit in China. It was reported from Hong Kong that the father, son, and daughter got H5N1 avian influenza. There was a concern that the illness in this [Canadian] family might be avian influenza. We were also concerned about measles since there were several cases of measles in Toronto at that time.

On Wednesday, I was in Kingston giving a talk on polio. I got a call from Dr. Michael Finkelstein [another associate medical officer of health in Toronto] that the family members did not have TB. He asked me to take on the investigation of the family who may have influenza as he was dealing with the measles outbreak.

I took the train back from Kingston to Toronto. I wasn't sure what the young man had since he didn't have TB and other family members were ill. I was trying to arrange for negative pressure rooms in hospitals. The family members, a brother, sister, and wife, were in three separate hospitals. The family had emigrated from Hong Kong to Canada eight years previously. The mother had recently died at home.

We had some language difficulties getting a detailed story from some family members but eventually found out that the mom and dad had visited a son in Hong Kong. After they returned, the mother became ill and sought advice from her family doctor. The doctor told her to stay home and that she had a "viral" illness. She worsened at home and died several days later. The coroner investigated and determined she probably had had a myocardial infarction, or heart attack. This was noted on the death certificate with an underlying viral illness. The picture wasn't clear. It certainly wasn't what we thought it was.

Eighteen hours after he had initially come to the hospital, the son was put in a negative pressure room. The son worsened and died on Thursday. By the end of the day, his brother was in the ICU. His wife and son were also ill and in the hospital as was his sister.

A few days later, the father also got sick. He was a poor historian and was unclear about the trip to Hong Kong, so we went to the house and found luggage tags, and from those, we determined the travel itinerary.

A press release by public health and the involved hospitals on Friday told everyone about the family so we could identify contacts. A large number of people had been to the mom's funeral. Two brothers were sick, and one had died. There were more than 600 contacts of the family members identified in the first day.

I was still thinking it was influenza. There were alerts about a similar illness in Hong Kong. We were trying to find contacts. In the middle of the next week, a health care worker in a hospital emergency room became ill. We didn't know what it was.

Around the 21st or 22nd, I was working with two other epidemiologists including Dr. Allison McGeer, an infectious disease specialist at Mount Sinai Hospital. We went out and got lists of all the hospital staff to try and figure out who was sick. We developed a questionnaire to figure out what was going on. We initially found nine people. Over the next 48 hours, we found 9, then 11, then 13, then 15 people who were ill. We realized that people were incubating this disease longer than we had thought.

From March 23rd to the 25th, we closed the hospital. Completely closed. We opened an isolation ward in the old TB hospital for the staff members to go. It was very tough. They were being separated from their spouses and children. We implemented a work quarantine and isolated people who were not ill but who were contacts of those who were ill.

All the hospitals are publicly funded, but they are privately run. They have their own boards. The government has a stewardship role. I notified the CEO of the hospital that something was going on. I worked closely with the Ontario Ministry of Health and notified them. We worked closely in closing the initial affected hospital.

Dr. Colin d'Cunha was the chief medical officer for the province of Ontario. He notified Tony Clement, who was the minister of health for Ontario.

Mayor Lastman was notified. John Fillion, the city councillor who was the chair of the Board of Health for the City of Toronto, was notified. The mayor, to his credit, said, "Do what you need to do."

Around the second week, a lot of things happened at the hospital and the crisis got a lot bigger.

The city's emergency operations center [EOC] was activated. The emergency committee met every second day for the first six weeks. We would brief them early in the morning around 6:30 to 7 A.M. The committee was chaired by the deputy mayor, Case Ootes. It included police, fire, city works, Emergency Medical Services, the office of Emergency Management, and other city leaders. We, TPH, took the lead, and they supported us. We kept the political people and the EOC informed. It worked well at the city level.

On March 26, Dr. Sheela Basrur, Toronto medical officer of health, and I went to the provincial EOC. Dr. Jim Young, the commissioner of public security, was in charge of the provincial response. The premier then declared a provincial public health emergency. Once that was declared, provincial and federal resources became available. We're much stronger at the provincial level than individual states in the United States are, but we are weaker at the federal level than the United States.

At the first meeting at the provincial EOC, Sheela and I attended a meeting with the premier who said, "Do whatever you need to do to stop this." Both the premier and minister of health were briefed daily. They were involved in decision making. I thought they had a very appropriate level of involvement. The premier deferred to the medical and public health experts and said, "I'm not a physician. I need you to make the decisions." They didn't interfere, which I think is a good thing. It is important to define the public role of politicians. This was clearly a public health and medical crisis that needed to be handled by people who had the expertise to do so.

For the most part, press briefings were done by the public health people and infectious disease physicians who were able to talk knowledgeably about what was happening and provide appropriate advice to the public. The elected officials were not as visible with the press. But from the inside, they were very involved. They intentionally left it to public health. SARS was a very complex medical situation.[19]

CONCLUSION

If misunderstandings exist between political and public health leaders, then responses to crises such as epidemics and bioterrorist attacks can be jeopardized. For an effective response, public health officials need political support and elected officials need public health support. Elected officials, unless they plan to take on the roles and responsibilities of public health professionals during times of crisis, must appoint competent, qualified professionals who are able to handle the challenges of epidemics or bioterrorist attacks.

All crises, especially if they disrupt normal societal functioning, are inherently political. However, depending on the personalities and leadership qualities of the individuals involved, the political leader may prefer to control decision making, rather than delegate it to the professional appointee. In essence, there could be two models of crisis leadership: the Giuliani Model, in which the political leader makes the decisions with expert advice, or the Glendening Model, in which the public health leader makes the decisions with the political leader's support.

The case studies profiled in this chapter illustrate that the public health leaders most effective in responding to the crises were the ones working in robust public health and medical systems with good working relationships with political leaders. During the anthrax crisis in New Jersey, DiFerdinando ran into difficulties because the state did not have a well-integrated public health and medical system: he was forced to recommend that postal workers obtain antibiotics from their private physicians after CDC officials refused to release antibiotics from the National Strategic Stockpile. He was in the unfortunate position of being an acting health commissioner working with an acting governor. They did not have time to develop a relationship before the crisis hit, resulting in DiFerdinando's making decisions without political support.

In the United States, both the Giuliani and Glendening models are in use; in Canada, with its parliamentary system, the Glendening Model appears to prevail. Clear division of responsibilities between parliament and the executive branch characterizes European governments as well, whereas in the United States, these roles are fragmented. In the United States, elected officials often play a much larger role in the implementation of public policy.[20] This blurring of roles between politicians and bureaucrats might contribute to leadership confusion during a crisis. Leadership problems can arise if the elected officials and the experts do not understand what each expects from the other.

Some individuals, given their unique personalities and leadership qualities, would be best served to employ one model rather than another. For example, New York City Health Commissioner Cohen preferred his role as an advisor to Mayor Giuliani. In contrast, Dr. Georges Benjamin, the secretary of health in Maryland, was happy to take the lead with the political support of Governor Glendening.

The founders of the United States designed the government so that no one individual would accumulate too much power. This was an important design feature that was meant to help ensure that no tyrant or dictator would emerge in the future. Public authority is deliberately and institutionally fragmented and shared.[21] The consequences of dividing responsibility and accountability might be a government system inherently less robust at responding to crises than other types of democracies. The end result is that, in the United States, the success or failure of a public health crisis response is largely dependent on the individual political and public health leaders involved.

In Canada, the public health and medical professionals made decisions with political support. According to Dr. Henry, the political leaders provided support but didn't communicate with the media. Instead, they deferred to the experts to communicate. Even though this strategy worked in that the epidemic was eventually contained, the media and the public perceived the political leaders as uninvolved and weak.

What is clear from these case studies is that public health and political leadership are equally important during infectious disease crises. The political leaders decide how much decision-making authority they will delegate to the professionals. Their relationships with their appointees must be based on mutual respect and trust.

Chapter 6

CONFRONTING UNCERTAINTY

In the spring of 1997, the avian influenza A (H5N1) virus jumped the species barrier and began infecting humans in Hong Kong. In May, a three-year-old boy became sick and died. In total, 18 people became ill and were hospitalized. Six died. Despite scientific questions about the new virus, significant economic implications, and enormous logistical challenges, authorities proceeded to cull more than a million chickens to control the outbreak. Some experts believe that the slaughter averted an imminent human pandemic.

Although all crises begin with uncertainty and confusion, disease outbreaks, such as avian influenza A, create unique challenges for leaders. New outbreaks combine the threat of immediate, wide-scale harm—demanding a swift response—with a degree of scientific complexity that usually requires lengthy research and analysis to understand. Leaders are forced to take action even though action brings its own risks.

This chapter describes some of the challenges leaders face when confronting new disease threats. In some cases, scientific information can be ambiguous, incomplete, or unavailable. Influenza A generates considerable concern because the virus is always mutating and previous pandemics in 1918, 1957, and 1968 were deadly. Three influenza A crises illustrate the difficult decisions that leaders must make when a new virus emerges. The 2009 influenza A H1N1 crisis demonstrates that global hysteria and inappropriate government policies can develop despite early warning and advances in scientific knowledge.

Four expert scientists were asked how leaders should handle these situations. Even with expert scientific advice, leaders must use their best judgment and common sense when making tough decisions.

THE 1976–77 SWINE FLU DILEMMA

In January 1976, an outbreak of influenza at Fort Dix, New Jersey, caused one death, 13 hospitalizations, and an estimated 230 cases of a novel strain of a flu virus.[1] At that time, it was known that the 1918 pandemic had been caused by an H1N1-type influenza strain, and it was believed that the strain isolated in New Jersey was related to it.[2] However, it was not known if the newly identified strain of influenza would lead to the next killer pandemic.

On February 13, 1976, Dr. Edwin Kilbourne, a respected influenza specialist and chairman of the department of microbiology at the Mount Sinai School of Medicine in New York City, published an editorial in the *New York Times* stating that influenza pandemics had occurred exactly once every 11 years since the 1940s—and that the next pandemic was imminent. Kilbourne claimed that the United States should prepare for this natural disaster by establishing an advisory commission to coordinate the influenza-related research activities of the National Institute for Allergy and Infectious Diseases and by immunizing 45 million people, especially susceptible Americans.[3]

One week later, the *New York Times* reported that U.S. federal health experts were alerting all state health departments and the World Health Organization (WHO) that the virus that caused the 1918–19 pandemic might have returned. The Fort Dix virus was a hybrid between a human Asian flu virus and a virus that caused a flu-like illness in swine. Dr. Bruce Dull, assistant director of the U.S. Centers for Disease Control and Prevention (CDC) and Dr. Walter Dowdle of the CDC Virology Division noted that the current influenza vaccine would be useless during a pandemic and that it would take at least six months for a new effective vaccine to be produced.[4]

From February to March of that year, testing at Fort Dix suggested that as many as 500 soldiers had been infected by swine flu. The CDC was in a difficult position. If it did nothing and a pandemic emerged, millions of people would be clamoring for an unavailable or limited vaccine supply. If millions of doses of vaccine were made and a pandemic did not occur, it would be accused of wasting public money.[5] Dr. David Sencer, director of the CDC, convened the Advisory Committee on Immunization Practices (ACIP) in March to review the findings and decide on a course of action.[6]

The members of ACIP disagreed on how to proceed. Dr. Russell Alexander, a public health physician at the University of Washington School of Public Health, recommended stockpiling the vaccine rather than vaccinating 200 million people for a perceived, but unclear, threat. Others stressed that if there were a pandemic and deaths, and they had vaccine in refrigerators but could not get it to people in time, then they would be accused of doing nothing. In the end, the committee decided to proceed with vaccine production and develop a plan for its administration.[7]

Sencer wrote to the secretary of health, education and welfare (HEW), outlining the problem and presenting four courses of action: (1) do nothing, and rely on private health care providers to serve those who want vaccination; (2) a minimal response, limiting the government role to vaccinating traditional federal beneficiaries; (3) full-scale immunization of the entire U.S. population, carried out by the federal government and the public sector; and (4) a combined approach, in which the federal government would contract with private pharmaceutical companies to produce vaccines for the entire U.S. population but would distribute them to the public through a variety of channels, including private physicians.[8]

Sencer recommended the fourth option, arguing that "the Administration can tolerate unnecessary health expenditures better than unnecessary death and illness if a pandemic should occur."[9] Unfortunately, Sencer's advice was misrepresented. A HEW staff member sent a memo to the White House comparing the current situation to the 1918 pandemic that had killed between 20 and 40 million people worldwide. Sencer had compared the swine flu situation to the less severe 1957–58 Asian and 1968–69 Hong Kong pandemics—not the deadly 1918 pandemic.[10]

By March 19, there were no new cases of influenza detected around Fort Dix.[11] Nonetheless, on March 24, President Gerald Ford met with a "blue-ribbon" panel of experts, including Drs. Jonas Salk, Albert Sabin, Edwin Kilbourne, and David Sencer to hear the CDC proposal and make recommendations. After the meeting, President Ford announced that he accepted the CDC recommendations and launched the National Influenza Immunization Program (NIIP).[12] The House and Senate passed an appropriations bill for $137 million to purchase vaccines that Ford signed into law on April 15, 1976. In October of that year, the first swine flu shots were administered.[13]

The NIIP immunized 45 million people in 10 weeks. Even though the vaccines appeared safe during initial trials, the program received two damaging blows: the first when vaccine manufacturers demanded that the government indemnify them against claims of adverse reactions, leading the public to believe that "there's something wrong with the vaccine."[14]

The second blow occurred when approximately 944 cases of Guillain-Barré syndrome, an adverse reaction, developed among vaccine recipients and received considerable coverage by the press.[15] As the number of these adverse reactions increased, Sabin—one of President Ford's blue-ribbon experts—claimed in the *New York Times* that the CDC was using scare tactics when it compared the current swine flu to the 1918 pandemic and was destroying public trust in the process.[16] He wrote that the March decision to prepare for a potential pandemic was prudent, but that the situation had changed when no additional cases were detected at home or abroad. He believed that to continue to recommend the vaccine was both reckless and futile: any vaccine administered in that flu season would be useless against a future pandemic.[17]

In the end, the swine flu pandemic never materialized.

The reputation of the leaders responding to the swine flu outbreak was further tarnished on December 21, 1976, when Harry Schwartz, a member of the editorial board of the *New York Times,* wrote in an article titled, "Swine Flu Fiasco":

> Last February and March, on the flimsiest of evidence, President Ford and the Congress were panicked into believing that the country stood at the threshold of a killer pandemic. . . . Today, there is no sign whatsoever of anything approaching a swine flu epidemic; but . . . the millions of dollars of federal money spent and the vast vaccination program . . . may have resulted in the death of some persons and sickened many more.[18]

The swine flu outbreak and the subsequent response of leaders provided many lessons. In 1977, Joseph Califano, Jr., secretary of the U.S. Department of Health, Education and Welfare wrote:

> The swine flu experience threw into sharp relief two questions that increasingly challenge officials at the high policy levels of government: First, how shall top lay officials, who are not themselves expert, deal with fundamental policy questions that are based, in part, on highly technical and complex expert knowledge—especially when that knowledge is speculative, or hotly debated, or when "the facts" are so uncertain? Second, how should policymakers—and their expert advisers—seek to involve and educate the public and relevant parties on such complicated and technical issues?[19]

In January 2006, Dr. Richard Krause, director of the National Institute of Allergy and Infectious Diseases from 1975 to 1984, characterized the uncertainty surrounding any infectious disease outbreak as analogous to the fog of war and cautioned scientists and public health professionals to base their crisis response decisions on expert opinion and their own evaluation of the facts.[20]

In his own reflections on the swine flu program, Sencer indicated that the prevailing perception was that the response was motivated by politics rather than by science and that President Ford's highly publicized meeting with scientists amplified this perception. Instead, Sencer believed that communication would have been more effective if it had come to the public from scientifically qualified individuals:[21]

Swine flu occurred during an election year. It became a presidential initiative in the White House, and the press became suspicious that it was a political issue. It would have been much better if the White House had not staged a large public relations event. The White House insisted that both Albert Sabin and Jonas Salk attend a meeting to discuss the situation. Neither was an expert in influenza epidemiology or virology. The meeting was followed by a formal press conference with Albert and Jonas beside the President. This set the stage for the entire program to be considered a political move rather than an attempt to protect the public. It became a media and political event.

When politicians begin speaking as experts in science without regard to scientific advice, there is trouble. Instead, they should use scientists as spokespersons for science. This person must be able to answer questions. Over time, there has been a trend of politicians assuming those roles rather than staying with the policy aspects.

During the swine flu program, we brought together divergent opinions. There was general consensus except for one dissenter. Yet on television he got equal time compared to the spokesman for the opinion of all 49 other states. It was equal time but not necessarily equal weight.

Leadership by committee doesn't work. Committees should be used for advice, but not to make decisions.

Ultimately, the policy leader must make the final decision and take responsibility for what happens. The protection of the public should be the top priority. All policy decisions entail risks and benefits: risks or benefits to the decision maker; risks or benefits to those affected by the decision. I believe, unfortunately, that in today's political climate, the risks to the decision maker too frequently are put first.[22]

THE 1997 AVIAN FLU DILEMMA

Twenty years later, public health officials faced a more daunting influenza virus: the avian influenza A (H5N1) virus.[23] This new virus first gained attention in 1997 when wild waterfowl began transmitting the virus to domestic poultry and, eventually, to humans in Hong Kong.[24] Eighteen humans who had contact with living or recently killed birds were initially hospitalized, but subsequent victims began appearing in November and December.[25]

Early in December, Dr. Margaret Chan, Hong Kong's director of health, invited local and foreign flu experts to investigate the outbreak.[26] After an emergency meeting, they issued guidelines to all physicians on how to treat potential bird flu patients. Dr. Saw Thian-aun, deputy director of the Hong Kong health department, said that a vaccine against the virus was being developed. Tung Chee-hwa, Hong Kong's chief executive and principal political leader, urged Hong Kong residents not to panic.[27]

On December 17, Hong Kong's health, agriculture, and hospital officials met to develop strategies to prevent further spread. The committee ordered enhanced disease surveillance in both poultry and humans, tighter import controls on chickens, and improvements in environmental hygiene in the live animal markets. Chickens outside of Hong Kong would have to be certified as virus free by Chinese veterinarians.[28]

Because almost 75 percent of all chickens sold in Hong Kong were from mainland China, Lessie Wei Chi Kit-yee, Agriculture and Fisheries director, encouraged officials in Guangzhou Province to increase their surveillance of diseased birds. To reduce widespread fear, Anson Chan Fang On-sang, the chief secretary for the administration, announced an interdepartmental task force to keep the public informed, and the health department established two hotlines to provide information to the public.[29]

At a Hong Kong Farmers' Association meeting on December 20, farmers reported that they were no longer able to feed their flocks because the public stopped buying chickens: business had dropped by 70 percent. Farmers recommended that millions of their chickens be slaughtered and requested that the Hong Kong government compensate them for these losses. The Agriculture and Fisheries Department responded that the move was unnecessary because most of the chickens were from mainland China.[30]

As the crisis continued, hostilities developed among the government, chicken sellers, and the media. Chief Executive Tung complained privately that the media had stoked the public's fears and reduced tourism. Yuen Ka-chai, president of the International Chinese Tourist Association, also accused the press of paying too much attention to the issue. Chicken sellers attacked reporters in the animal markets, accusing them of exaggerating the problem and ruining their business. The press accused government officials of not being open and transparent during the early stages of the crisis.[31]

On December 29, Stephen Ip, secretary for economic services, announced that 1.2 million chickens would be slaughtered in an effort to contain the spread of the disease, and that farmers would be compensated for their losses. The decision was made after health officials discovered bird flu virus in samples taken from Hong Kong's largest poultry market.

As many as 2,000 workers from seven different government departments and agencies were to gas, sterilize (to neutralize the virus, which can still be infectious even when the bird is dead), and bury all poultry, including ducks and geese, in 1,000 markets and 160 farms, in 24 hours. All chickens imported from mainland China were banned.[32]

Slaughtering more than a million birds was more difficult than expected. Most workers had no experience handling birds or administering gas and lacked sufficient protective clothing. There were not enough suitable carbon dioxide gas cylinders.[33] Many chickens escaped the slaughter and were found wandering through farms and housing developments. Plastic sacks of dead chickens lay unburied along roadsides; dogs, cats, and rats ate through bags and carried carcasses away. Government officials found almost 70 farms that had not participated in the slaughter.[34]

One editorial stated that:

> Rightly or wrongly, there is a widespread perception of a lack of leadership during this crisis. . . . there must be clear and visible indications that Mr. Tung and senior aides are in charge.[35]

Despite problems with leadership and logistics, some experts believe that the slaughter may have averted an imminent human pandemic.[36] The virus did not reappear in humans again until six years later in the Fujian Province of China.[37]

Since that time, the virus has become entrenched among poultry flocks in parts of Africa, Asia, and likely the Middle East.[38] Despite the spread among domestic birds, however, infections among humans remain relatively rare: as of June 2009, a total of 433 people have become ill from the virus since 2003.[39] Furthermore, although the global fear has been that the virus may develop the ability to infect humans easily (thus triggering the next deadly pandemic), the vast majority of cases have been caused by handling sick or dead poultry a week before the onset of illness.[40]

Political leaders must protect against a human pandemic whenever a disease jumps from animals to humans. But they must also consider the many government agencies and private sector businesses that can block a response if it runs counter to their interests. If an outbreak involves food-producing animals, such as poultry for example, then the decision to cull such animals raises trade and economic concerns and may be opposed by the agriculture community.

As of June 2009, Indonesia has had more human cases and deaths (141 and 115 respectively) from avian flu than any other country since 2003.[41] There is evidence that this is a direct result of decisions made by agriculture, not health, officials.

Indonesia has the largest population of humans and poultry in South-east Asia. According to Dr. Tri Satya Putri Naipospos, national director of Indonesia's animal health and a respected animal health expert, Indonesian agriculture officials knew of avian influenza in the country's poultry populations since the middle of 2003, but they kept this knowledge secret because of heavy lobbying by the poultry industry. Naipospos repeated her allegations in *Kompas,* an influential local newspaper, and was subsequently fired by the Agriculture Ministry.[42]

By the time Indonesia confirmed its avian influenza outbreak in January 2004, the virus had already spread across Java to the Bali and Sumatra islands.[43] Instead of culling all poultry near the outbreak (as recommended by the UN Food and Agriculture Organization), Indonesian officials decided to vaccinate their birds. Their vaccination efforts were below the threshold required for effectiveness, however, and as the virus spread in poultry, it increasingly crossed the species barrier to infect humans.[44]

Alan Sipress was a foreign correspondent for the *Washington Post* based in Jakarta, Indonesia, from 2002 to 2006 and closely followed the avian flu outbreak in Asia:

> In much of the third world and Asia, departments of agriculture are much more powerful than [departments of] health. The reason for this is that agriculture makes up substantial parts of these countries' economies. Issues about food availability are very important. In controversies that pit health against agriculture, agriculture always wins. This is especially the case in China.
>
> The agriculture folks were covering up avian influenza in birds. For an exporting country, there was huge economic pressure not to cut off exports. For example, Thailand was the fourth largest international exporter of chickens to the rest of the world with huge exports to Europe. In January 2004, the virus was spreading in Thai poultry for two months, but it was not announced. People were saying it was fowl plague or Newcastle disease. On January 19, 2004, Thai officials told the European Union Consumer Protection Commissioner David Byrne that there was no bird flu in Thailand. Four days later on January 23, 2004, Thai government officials confirmed its outbreaks, and the Europeans went ballistic and cut off imports.
>
> Indonesia doesn't export much, but it has a huge domestic market. It has been a democracy since 1998 when Suharto was overthrown. The ministers are drawn from different political parties. There were a number of problems between Dr. Naipospos [the former national director of animal health] and the agriculture minister, who comes from a moderate Islamist party. His is an appointed position, but it is a very political position.
>
> [Naipospos] was telling the truth and criticizing the ministry. She had two strikes against her: she was a Christian and a woman. The health minister is a woman too. There were a number of personal dynamics at work. The

bird flu outbreak in Indonesia was covered up for six months and then ignored for eighteen months. The virus is now endemic in that country.[45]

THE 2009 SWINE FLU DILEMMA

Thirty-three years after the 1976–77 swine flu virus crisis, a second swine flu virus emerged generating global panic. In mid-March 2009, Mexican health officials began receiving reports of influenza-like illnesses in parts of the country. Surveillance efforts intensified after April 17 when a case of atypical (unusual) pneumonia was reported in Oaxaca State. However, these enhanced surveillance efforts focused on severely ill hospitalized patients rather than on the general community so the reported death rates were spuriously high.[46] Much of the Mexican population lacks health insurance, so people prefer to self-medicate rather than seek medical care.[47] Mexico quickly notified the Pan American Health Organization (PAHO), the regional office for the Americas of the World Health Organization, of the new influenza outbreak in accordance with the new international health regulations.[48] Mexico's initial reports of high death rates likely contributed to global fears that a new influenza killer had emerged.

At the end of March, the CDC received reports of two children in Southern California who had influenza-like illnesses. The children had not been exposed to swine nor had they traveled to Mexico. There was no contact between them yet they both tested positive for a new influenza A (H1N1) virus. The virus, which had been circulating in swine since 1998, contained re-assorted avian, human, and swine genes. It was also the same virus that was infecting people in Mexico.[49]

On April 25, Mexican president Felipe Calderon assumed emergency powers to isolate people infected with the virus. Despite risking severe economic and political consequences, Mexican officials shut businesses, canceled concerts, closed museums, banned spectators from attending two soccer matches, and closed schools in and around Mexico City for over a week in an attempt to contain the outbreak.[50] WHO declared the new virus a public health emergency of international concern. The next day, the United States declared a public health emergency, and on April 29, WHO raised the pandemic influenza phase from four to five.[51]

Unfortunately, the United States did not have national health leaders in place to address the crisis. Almost 100 days into the new administration, Senate Republicans were still stalling the approval of Kansas governor Kathleen Sebelius, President Barack Obama's choice for secretary of the Department of Health and Human Services, because of her record of supporting abortion rights. The CDC still lacked a permanent director. Indeed, many of the top health positions remained unfilled. Janet Napolitano, the secretary of the Department of Homeland Security, and an acting CDC director filled the void.[52] Increasing public pressure prompted the Senate to confirm Governor Sebelius on April 28.[53]

Other countries responded quickly, but not necessarily appropriately. While Mexican leaders made difficult decisions to stem the outbreak, other countries, in response, unfairly targeted Mexican citizens and businesses. The Chinese sent health officials clad in biohazard suits onto planes arriving from Mexico and the United States to haul off Mexican nationals into forced quarantine.[54] China, Russia, the Philippines, and other nations banned pork products from Mexico and some parts of the United States in the mistaken belief that pork consumption transmitted the virus.

The Egyptians slaughtered 300,000 healthy pigs even though there wasn't a single case of swine flu in the country. Egypt's Coptic Christian minority accused the government leaders of using swine flu fears to unfairly punish them economically. Most of the pig farmers in Egypt belong to the minority Coptic Christian population since the Muslim majority doesn't eat pork because of religious restrictions.[55]

In response, World Health officials decided to rename the swine flu crisis the "2009 H1N1 virus outbreak" in order to stop countries from inappropriately banning pork products and slaughtering pigs.[56] The World Animal Health Organization strongly advised against these policies since there was no evidence that live swine or pork products were involved in the epidemic.[57]

Attempting to calm the public's fears, U.S. president Barack Obama stated that the flu was a "cause for deep concern but not panic." Obama's efforts to reassure the nation, however, were thwarted by Vice President Joseph Biden. During an interview on NBC's *Today* show, Biden stated that he would advise his family not to travel anywhere in aircraft or other confined places. His comments generated anger particularly from transportation industries, especially the airlines. Richard E. Besser MD, the acting director of the CDC, reminded the public that seasonal flu caused, on average, 36,000 deaths per year.[58]

As the epidemic progressed, health officials discovered that the virus appeared only slightly more contagious and no deadlier than seasonal flu, and they subsequently recommended that schools reopen. On May 4, Mexican officials lowered their public health alert and stated that they would allow most businesses to reopen later in the week.[59]

The disease continued to spread. Despite the generally mild illnesses, China increased its vigilance and virtually imprisoned several thousand foreigners and Chinese nationals into quarantine facilities even if they had minor signs and symptoms such as slightly elevated temperatures, coughs, or sniffles. The Chinese policies antagonized other countries. Mexico chartered a plane to bring its nationals home after accusing China of targeting its citizens.[60]

The benign pandemic required public health leaders to rethink how to address disease severity. Unlike the Chinese officials who maintained draconian measures, leaders in the Americas and Europe revised their policies to reflect the reduced severity of the disease.

WHO officials decided not to elevate the pandemic classification to phase six, the highest level signifying sustained disease transmission in general populations, until June 11 because they were concerned that the "pandemic" designation would generate even more global hysteria.[61] However, by that time, 74 countries had already reported the virus in 28,774 laboratory-confirmed cases including 144 deaths. Mexico reported 108 deaths—more than any other country.[62]

Scientists examining the 2009 swine flu virus's genome found that it lacked virulence markers, such as a key DNA sequence coding for a protein called PB1-F2 that the deadly pandemic influenza viruses of 1918, 1957, and 1968 possessed. The avian influenza A (H5N1) virus also had this virulence marker but lacked the ability to spread easily from person-to-person.[63] Peter Palese, chairman of the department of microbiology at the Mount Sinai School of Medicine and a top influenza expert, wrote an opinion piece in the *Wall Street Journal* about the virus in an attempt to allay public fears.[64] Unfortunately, despite the advances in deciphering the virus's genetic make-up, scientists have been unable to predict if the 2009 swine flu virus will acquire virulence factors in the future.[65] As of the writing of this book, the 2009 swine flu pandemic continues to spread.

LEADERS' RESPONSES TO DISEASE THREATS

Because disease outbreaks can wreak havoc on affected countries' economies, it is perhaps understandable that political and bureaucratic leaders would want to deny that a problem exists in order to maintain economic and social stability. However, denial may lead to a far worse situation than if the outbreak is readily acknowledged and rapidly confronted.

China's leaders have a history of ignoring or downplaying disasters because they believe these events reflect poorly on their political legitimacy.[66] Between 2002 and 2003, China denied the existence of Severe Acute Respiratory Syndrome (SARS) for four months and then subsequently hindered outbreak investigations. As a result of these decisions, SARS struck 26 countries, sickened over 8,000 people and killed almost 800 by July 2003.[67] With its credibility destroyed and economy hit hard, China demonstrated how not to respond to an infectious disease crisis.[68]

How should leaders respond to deadly outbreaks? What information is needed to make rational decisions? Four senior scientists were asked how leaders should approach crises in which the fundamental scientific knowledge is unclear or unknown.

From 1974 to 1988, Dr. Thomas Monath led the CDC Laboratory for Vector-Borne Diseases. He subsequently became chief of virology at the U.S. Army Medical Research Institute for Infectious Diseases, where he focused on vaccines and antiviral medications against insect-borne viral diseases.[69] After working at the pharmaceutical company Acambis, Monath became a partner with Kleiner, Perkins, Caufield & Byers to lead their pandemic and biodefense fund.[70] Here are his thoughts on dealing with a public health crisis:

> The first issue is always diagnosis. There should be a pre-event infrastructure with centralized genomics databases, strain and reagent repositories, diagnostic testing expertise, and so on. Unfortunately, we are worse off in some areas [of preparedness] such as the underfunded arbovirus[71] research center at the [University of Texas, Medical Branch] than earlier.
>
> There should be pre-positioned field investigation teams with different specialties/competencies ready to go on short notice. Clarification requires on-site investigation. There should be emergency measures in place to move teams and specimens—there should be no red tape.
>
> Experts in different syndromes and diseases should be identified in advance. Leaders should rapidly convene panels to study the problem at hand and provide advice. There should be memorandums of understanding and cooperative agreements in place between different agencies to reduce response times and improve efficiencies. This is in place for bioterrorism, but not for public health emergencies.
>
> There should be public health staff in all embassies who could develop relationships with health ministries at the diplomatic level. We should be supporting field research programs to study transmission cycles of viruses in wild animals. Remote sensing, which might provide critical information, could be applied and interpreted quickly.
>
> Decisions should be based on scientific evidence, advice/consensus of expert advisory panels, and agency personnel, in a coordinated way. It is important to inform the public of the process and demonstrate that all stakeholders are represented in decision making. When an event involves more than one country, or has the potential to spread, it is obvious to involve WHO and other countries' health agencies to reach consensus on a plan of action.
>
> The planning for avian influenza is the best model. This is the best case scenario because there has been time to prepare. Avian influenza has been approached by international agencies and individual countries. [We should] evaluate how well this advanced planning stands up in the event a pandemic occurs.

Politicians/administrators would make the decisions, but they should be based on all available evidence from the scientific community. In the United States, the Department of Health and Human Services would make recommendations to the White House with transparency and clarification that the best minds outside of government have been consulted.[72]

Dr. Lawrence (Larry) Kerr is the senior bio advisor in the National Counterproliferation Center, U.S. Office of the Director of National Intelligence. From 2001 to 2006, Kerr served in the White House Office of Science and Technology Policy and the Homeland Security Council as the director for biodefense policy.

The terrorist events of 2001 have clearly shaped how we view an infectious disease outbreak within the United States or anywhere in the world. In the absence of data, we assume that any disease outbreak (in humans, animals, or plants) could be a potential biological attack until proven otherwise. What this means in the real world is that there is now a much closer working relationship between the public health sectors and the scientific, law enforcement, and responder communities at all levels—federal, state, local, tribal, and private.

These communities have a much greater awareness of one another's capabilities; they train, exercise, and prepare for an all-hazard response—whether the public health threat is made by humans or nature. Take, for example, when SARS first appeared on the international scene in late 2002/early 2003, we speculated that the outbreak was worse than what China was telling the world through the media. Isolated cases were spreading to cities outside of China, and there was a 6–12 week period when we didn't know what the pathogen was. It could have been a natural pathogen, a laboratory accident, or a potential biowarfare agent.

In February 2003, when Canada recognized that it had patients with symptoms of SARS, the fact that suddenly the pathogen was much closer to home was a real wake-up call within the United States.

Even once the virus was identified in April 2003, there were early reports from the DNA sequencing of the viral SARS genome that suggested there might have been a sequence similar to that found in some commercial vectors commonly used in molecular biology labs. This initially caused some concern because it may have been the indication that this pathogen was human-made.

Fortunately, additional sequencing of other SARS isolates did not have this sequence, and its similarity to the other coronovirus family members demonstrated that it was most probably from a natural reservoir. There was clearly a significant period of time when we simply did not have all the available information to determine whether SARS was a deliberate or human-made infectious agent. Despite this knowledge, public health officials used a variety of measures to minimize the outbreak and ultimately contain it.

Based on the sheer number and diversity of pathogens in nature—and there are so many pathogens about which we know so little—there is going to be a time delay in our ability to give the ground truth to policymakers about a disease outbreak. Although groundbreaking medical technologies are in development and making it to the clinic and bedside, we are often faced with one limiting step—the isolation and ability to grow the pathogen before we can seek to identify and characterize it. Sometimes to get the answers, you have to wait until the experimental results are finished and interpreted. It is very unsatisfying to give speculative answers or to have to answer "we just don't know" to decision makers—but events such as the aforementioned have sensitized the public and the policymakers to the inherent uncertainties regarding the life sciences.[73]

Dr. Jean-Claude Manuguerra, DVM, is the director of the Laboratory for Urgent Response to Biological Threats, Institut Pasteur. He currently serves as chairman for the French Advisory Committee on Influenza.

If scientific data are unknown, decisions still have to be made. In the past, well-known scientists advised ministers or high-ranking officials on scientific matters. Personal connections were usually involved—somebody knew someone who could give advice. Everything changed after the French HIV blood scandal.[74] At that time, there was no scientific rationale for what was done. After the disaster surfaced, a special tribunal was set up to try the ministers because otherwise they had immunity from prosecution. The prime minister's career was essentially over. The minister of social affairs and national solidarity left political life.

Ministers used to contact one, two, or three famous scientists to give advice. Now, we have scientists with collective expertise in standing advisory groups that provide advice to the government. We seek representation of different disciplines in these groups. There are groups for avian influenza and for pandemic [human] influenza.

Other groups are independent of any agency and report directly to the minister of health. If an issue or controversy transects disciplines or agencies, then the advisory group is likely to be inter-ministerial and the head is the chief medical officer from the National Department of Health.

When a new disease emerges, such as SARS, we use the most relevant group to give advice. For example, the pandemic influenza group was quickly mobilized to address SARS. The very day WHO announced its global alert for SARS, our group met in two to three hours in Paris. We are fortunate that Paris is only two to three hours away from virtually all parts of France.

Groups typically have a maximum of 20 people with an average of about 10 to 12 per meeting. Since we seek diverse expertise in these groups, there are epidemiologists, clinicians, veterinarians, pediatricians, geriatricians, and scientists. We want people who are competent. They are not static groups—there is turnover, but membership can last for years.

Collective expertise is critical, especially if the scientific evidence is not sound or is limited. The thinner the evidence, the better it is to have different points of view. Also, it is important to have preexisting groups rather than to quickly assemble an expert panel to address some crisis. The problem with newly assembled groups is that people try to look good and push their hypotheses or agendas forward. It is important to avoid personal convictions. People need to know how to work with one another and that takes time.

Of course, advice is advice. It depends on who is giving it. People who represent an organization or industry might try to sway opinion to their organization's benefit. Too informal a group is not good either. Membership in most advisory committees is competitive and voluntary. There is a call for candidates and a selection committee is established. We are evolving to have as transparent a process as possible.[75]

Lord Robert May, professor of zoology at Oxford University, was the chief scientific advisor to the government of the United Kingdom, head of the UK Office of Science and Technology from 1995 to 2000, and president of the Royal Society from 2000 to 2005:

I inherited the BSE [Bovine Spongiform Encephalopathy] crisis when I became the [UK] chief scientific advisor (CSA). That was the time when it first became clear that BSE could infect humans. I would like to think that if I had been CSA earlier, I wouldn't have said that BSE wouldn't infect humans. But with 20/20 hindsight, it is easy to say what one would or wouldn't have done under such circumstances. The best scientific advice would have been, "We can't be sure."

I produced a set of policy guidelines under John Major, revised under Tony Blair, and then revised again. They were short and succinct: only three to four pages. The guidelines essentially say: (1) when you come across something unknown, you get the best scientists; (2) at the same time, make sure all the dissonant views are heard; (3) no one should be excluded because of a conflict of interest; (4) the substance of the meetings should not be confidential—recommendations and conclusions should be published or otherwise available for scrutiny; and (5) admit what isn't known.

Having guidelines doesn't necessarily mean that the civil service will respond to them, but having them helps. It is important to make absolutely clear what we know and don't know, but there is always political pressure to be reassuring. There is a beneficial placebo effect to help people feel better with reassurance. After all, until fairly recently in medical history, doctors couldn't do much for people anyway—other than project an air of confidence. But it is important to be honest.

In the majority of disease outbreaks, the science is well established. In these circumstances, it is fine to get good, competent scientists. You don't need to get a Nobel Laureate. But if a crisis moves beyond the established knowledge base, then you need to get world-class experts.

Some scientists are better than others. I like to use this rock-climbing analogy: There are some scientists who are the pioneers who put up the ropes and ladders. Competent scientists can climb up the ropes and add something. The elite class of scientists climbs the rocks without ropes or ladders.

It is clear-cut who is in charge in the UK, as in much of the EU [European Union]. This distinction is much less so in the United States. There is a distinction between the professional civil service—the permanent secretaries—who do not change with elections, and the ministers who get elected. The ministers make policy and the civil service executes the policy. Of course, in areas in which science determines policy, you need to have appointed experts. What to do with this advice is a political choice.[76]

INFORMATION REQUIRED FOR DECISION MAKING

Before decisions can be made to address a public health crisis, political and public health leaders need specific information on which to base their decisions.

First, the pathogen causing the crisis needs to be identified as soon as possible. In the case of SARS, scientists from laboratories in the United States, Canada, Germany, and Hong Kong collaborated to identify the novel coronavirus.[77]

Epidemiologists then need to determine how the pathogen is transmitted so that measures to curtail further spread can be implemented. For example, it is important to know if the pathogen is transmitted via airborne droplets, water, or food. During the SARS epidemic, most people were not very infectious after developing symptoms, and traditional public health measures (e.g., quarantine, isolation, and contact tracing) were effective in curtailing spread.[78] In contrast, influenza A is far more difficult to control because people can be infectious before showing symptoms.

The source of an outbreak needs to be identified. For example, SARS was a novel zoonotic disease that emerged from bats and spread to other exotic animals that people ate.[79] If a pathogen were to emerge from wildlife or domestic animals, decisions would have to be made regarding culling herds or flocks in an attempt to break disease transmission. If an outbreak originated from a laboratory accident, then measures would have to be taken to tighten laboratory safety and security.

An August 2007 outbreak of foot-and-mouth disease on two farms in the United Kingdom was caused by a laboratory leak from either Merial (a corporate laboratory) or the Institute for Animal Health (a government animal health laboratory). The foot-and-mouth virus, which causes disease in livestock, is believed to have escaped from faulty wastewater systems that the two laboratories shared. The outbreak's economic impact was estimated at more than $100 million.[80]

The severity and spread of the disease must also be determined. Draconian measures would be more easily justified and accepted if the disease were deadly and contagious. For example, Hong Kong officials could justify culling all the poultry because the avian influenza A virus was lethal and was spreading. In contrast, after health officials realized that the 2009 swine flu virus was not deadly, they could not justify continuing strict containment measures.

Contact tracing must be done to identify individuals with possible exposure to the pathogen. Depending on the mode of transmission, infectiousness of the pathogen, and incubation period,[81] these individuals might be considered candidates for quarantine. In the case of pandemic influenza, however, quarantine is typically not effective because, as previously mentioned, asymptomatic people can be infectious.[82] For novel pathogens, a reliable and sensitive screening test should be developed and made available as soon as possible.

Similarly, people with symptoms associated with an outbreak should be identified with a reliable and sensitive diagnostic test—assuming one is available. If an effective treatment exists, decisions regarding its distribution would have to be made. Funding would be necessary for screening, hospitalization, and treatment. Countries in which universal access to medical care is *not* available would be at a disadvantage because the uninsured would likely delay treatment, thus inadvertently fanning disease spread.

Ideally, a safe and effective vaccine would be developed, produced, stockpiled, and administered as necessary. Developing a vaccine requires access to the causative agent, however, and if an outbreak originated in a developing country, cooperation in sharing the pathogen with the international community should not be assumed. Indonesian leaders, for example, refused to share samples of the avian influenza A virus with WHO because they believed that rich nations would develop vaccines for their own benefit and not share them. They wanted assurances that the vaccines would be available and affordable for developing countries.[83] Although their concerns were not unreasonable, their refusal to share viral samples potentially jeopardized global public health.

CONCLUSION

Political leaders, particularly those without an understanding of science, might find it difficult to make policy decisions when facing a deadly outbreak. Even with the advice of a committee of experts, decisions can be difficult because the experts might disagree, the scientific evidence might be unclear or unavailable, and/or response options might be controversial. Even for experts, scientific literature might be inconclusive or difficult to interpret.[84] In the end, leaders must rely on their best judgment and common sense when making decisions, especially when there is scientific uncertainty.

Regardless of who makes decisions, leaders must be aware that their decisions will be scrutinized for political motivation. For example, the decision to offer antibiotics or vaccines to one group of people but not another might be interpreted as discriminatory even if made with the best of intentions. Leaders have to make their decisions with the understanding that they have limited resources.

Leaders are frequently faulted for moving too slowly or too late to stop a disease crisis. During the initial stages of an outbreak, when the severity or spread is not apparent, however, it might be difficult to secure the political support needed to implement drastic measures. The 1976–77 swine flu episode illustrates what can happen when measures are implemented in a timely way in the face of a brewing crisis, but the crisis does not manifest. The leaders are then faulted for moving prematurely. On the other hand, Hong Kong leaders were faulted for moving too slowly in response to the avian influenza crisis.

Scientific advice is critical for effective decision making. The scientists interviewed for this chapter agreed that advice should be obtained from the best scientists and that decision making should be transparent. There must be an open discussion, ideally before a crisis develops, in which agreed-upon principles are applied to decisions. The public needs to know why and how decisions are made in order to get their support.

Political leaders must walk a fine line when deciding how to respond to an epidemic. However they decide to respond, they will run into great difficulties if they downplay the seriousness of the crisis or, worse, try to hide the crisis, as the Chinese leaders did during the early stages of the SARS outbreak.

The new international health regulations require nations to report outbreaks expeditiously so that containment measures can be promptly implemented. These new regulations are extremely important if an emerging disease crisis is deadly. However, a nation's disease surveillance and reporting capabilities are only as good as its medical and public health in frastructures. If initial reports are inaccurate, then inappropriate decisions might result.

Chapter 7

THE VITAL LINK BETWEEN ANIMAL AND HUMAN HEALTH

Part I

THE IMPACT OF ANIMAL HEALTH CRISES

In December 1984, a veterinarian was called to examine a cow suffering from poor coordination and an arched back on a farm in Sussex, England. Within months after the cow died, others on the farm began to show similar unusual signs before dying. By 1986, examination of brain samples from affected cattle demonstrated a new spongiform encephalopathy, and cattle on farms across England were showing signs of the same disease, prompting the British Central Veterinary Laboratory to draft a confidential communiqué, warning of the severe repercussions that the disease could potentially have on export trade and human life.

During the years that followed, the British government assembled a series of committees to provide advice on how to respond to *bovine spongiform encephalopathy* (BSE, otherwise known as *mad cow disease*). Experts concluded that the disease was most likely limited to cattle and focused on control of the means of transmission: contaminated animal feedstuff. However, critics accused the government of being too slow, limited, and opaque in its response, whether from a lack of information or a desire to protect the interests of food producers and the farming industry.

Identification of a new human condition, a variant Creutzfeldt-Jakob disease (vCJD) in 1996 and its epidemiological link to cattle BSE came just as control measures (restrictions on the use of certain cattle-derived proteins) were curtailing the cattle disease. Unfortunately, by 2003, the spread of the British mad cow disease epidemic was apparent: more than

180,000 cows were affected in countries across Europe and 143 people were diagnosed and died from vCJD.

The specter of an emerging zoonotic disease outbreak creates extraordinary challenges for leaders who must quickly decide how to respond while facing intense scrutiny from the media and the public. These challenges increase when the immediate threat to human life is unclear, which occurs when diseases such as BSE strike animal populations. Disease epidemics often emerge among animals before advancing to the human population, making them potentially lethal threats to humans and requiring input from scientific experts who are typically not involved in crisis management.

Throughout history, people have lived and worked alongside animals. Domesticated livestock and poultry provide food for humans. People also eat wild animals such as bison, deer, ducks, and rabbits; in some cultures, people eat exotic animals, such as apes, civet cats, and snakes. We keep pets in our homes and share the environment with wildlife. In developing countries, animals used for transport and farm animals often live alongside their owners.

The original mission of veterinary medicine was to ensure a stable food supply for people. In the 18th century, *rinderpest,* a deadly viral disease affecting cattle, devastated the human food supply. Pope Clement XI asked Dr. Giovanni Maria Lancisi, a physician, to combat the problem. Lancisi believed that rinderpest was communicable and recommended that all of the ill and suspect animals be killed and buried in lime. His novel concepts proved to be effective and are still widely practiced. The first school of veterinary medicine was established in Lyons, France, in 1762 to teach Lancisi's concepts.[1]

Three centuries later, society continues to suffer the consequences of animal disease epidemics. The outbreaks of BSE and foot-and-mouth disease (FMD) in livestock in the United Kingdom illustrate that animal disease outbreaks can lead to tremendous suffering and enormous economic costs and can impact public health. As with disease epidemics among human populations, effective leadership during animal disease epidemics is essential. Indeed, our reliance on animals for subsistence makes such leadership just as critical for the health and well-being of humans as it is during an outbreak of a deadly human disease.

Part I of this chapter describes the BSE crisis. Part II examines the foot-and-mouth (FMD) crisis. For both crises, leaders involved in the responses discuss their experiences.

BOVINE SPONGIFORM ENCEPHALOPATHY (BSE)

Although BSE is a recently recognized disease, *scrapie,* a similarly fatal and incurable neurodegenerative livestock disease, has been well known for 250 years. Since the 18th century, scrapie had been present in sheep herds in Great Britain.[2] In the late 1960s, its cause was still unknown; it was hypothesized to be a protein because it was minute and resisted measures that typically destroy DNA.[3] In 1982, Stanley Prusiner, a researcher at the University of California at San Francisco, proposed that the agent causing scrapie was an infectious protein that he called a *prion* (for "proteinaceous infectious particle").[4]

In addition to scrapie, prions have been linked to diseases in mink (transmissible mink encephalopathy) and deer (chronic wasting disease). Such diseases are not limited to animals, however. In humans, prions have been associated with several fatal neurodegenerative diseases, including Creutzfeldt-Jakob disease (CJD), Gerstmann-Straussler-Scheinker syndrome, and kuru. Although extremely rare, prion diseases can develop in a number of ways: spontaneously, through contact with infected individuals, or genetically.[5]

Before the 20th century, there was evidence that scrapie could spread from pregnant ewes to their unborn lambs and from sheep to sheep within a herd. There was also evidence that scrapie could exist in the environment (for example, in pastures) and spread disease.[6] But there was no reason to believe that it could cause disease in cattle or humans.

That began to change in 1984 when Dr. David Bee examined Cow 133, suffering from weight loss and an arched back on Pitsham Farm in Sussex, a county in southeast England.[7] Over a period of months, the cow began to lose coordination and to develop head tremors before dying on February 11, 1985. More cows on Pitsham Farm developed similar neurological signs before dying. Unsure of the cause, Bee and his colleagues sent another suffering cow (Cow 142) to the Central Veterinary Laboratory (CVL) in nearby Surrey for euthanasia and necropsy.

Carol Richardson, the pathologist at CVL, found spongiform changes in parts of the brain and spinal cord reminiscent of the changes seen with scrapie.[8] She sent the pathology samples and a copy of her report to Gerald Wells, head of the Neuropathology Section at CVL.

In September 1985, Wells reviewed Richardson's initial report of Cow 142 and examined the pathology samples of four other cows that had died on Pitsham Farm. Although he confirmed the pathological lesions, he concluded that a common cause could not be determined.

In late June 1986, however, spongiform encephalopathy was detected in a nyala[9] in a British wildlife park.[10] This was the first recognized case of a spongiform encephalopathy in a bovine species. One year after the nyala's death, the same wildlife park reported similar symptoms in a gemsbok, a different African antelope of a bovine species. There was no reported contact between the two animals.[11]

Cattle on other farms, such as the Plurenden Manor Farm in Kent, also began showing signs of the disease: nervousness, aggression, and inability to rise without assistance. Necropsies by the CVL of cows from farms in Bristol and Kent revealed signs of spongiform encephalopathy.[12]

On December 19, 1986, Ray Bradley, head of the CVL Pathology Department wrote to the CVL director of research and to Dr. William Watson, director of CVL, about the cases arriving from different farms, noting that their characteristics were similar to spongiform encephalopathies—particularly to scrapie in sheep:

> If the disease turned out to be bovine scrapie, it would have severe repercussions to the export trade and possibly also for humans if for example it was discovered that humans with spongiform encephalopathy had close association with the cattle. It is for these reasons that I have classified this document confidential.[13]

Although the memo was confidential, word spread about the possibility of a new infectious disease among cattle. In May 1987, Watson asked Dr. John Wilesmith, director of the CVL Epidemiology Unit, to investigate the new disease. Wilesmith began developing a database to track the cases and to investigate the etiology and spread of the disease that, by then, had been confirmed by examination of six cows from four farms.[14]

Barely one month later, however, William Howard Rees, chief veterinary officer of the Ministry of Agriculture, Fisheries and Food (MAFF) informed Donald Thompson, parliamentary secretary, that there was no evidence that the disease was transmissible to humans:

> Irresponsible or ill-informed publicity is likely to be unhelpful since it might lead to hysterical demands for immediate, draconian government measures and could lead other countries to reject UK export of live cattle and bovine embryos and semen. . . . The political implications of this development could be quite serious, particularly if not handled correctly.[15]

In response to Rees's memo, Sir Michael Franklin, the MAFF permanent secretary, held a meeting with Alistair Cruickshank, the MAFF undersecretary for animal health, Watson, and Rees. They agreed to publish a short factual report in the *Veterinary Record* (a publication of the British Veterinary Association) to ensure investigations were underway to assess possible links with human disorders, to provide a low-key scientific presentation at the British Cattle Veterinary Association, and to send a note to government ministers explaining the situation.[16]

At the end of September 1987, Derek Andrews succeeded Franklin as the MAFF permanent secretary. His appointment was accompanied by much greater visibility of the crisis: in October 1987, Wells published his findings of spongiform encephalopathy in cattle from dairy herds in the

Veterinary Record.[17] The *Sunday Telegraph* issued the first national newspaper report of an incurable disease wiping out dairy cattle.[18]

On March 3, 1988, Andrews contacted Sir Donald Acheson, chief medical officer of the UK Department of Health, for his advice on the potential risk of BSE to human health. Two weeks later, Acheson chaired a meeting that concluded that there was a need for an expert advisory panel on BSE; he informed the health ministers of the issue three days later and suggested Sir Richard Southwood, professor of zoology and pro vice-chancellor of Oxford University to head the group.[19]

The Southwood Working Party (SWP) was established in May 1988 and included Sir Anthony Epstein, a virologist at Wolfson College, Oxford University; Sir John Walton, professor of neurology, University of Newcastle-upon-Tyne; and Dr. William Martin, a veterinarian, formerly director of the Moredun Research Institute in Edinburgh. The group met in June 1988 to review the available BSE data and assess the possible implications for human health.[20]

During its first meeting, the SWP was concerned to discover that both healthy and BSE-affected animals were slaughtered and entered the food supply for human consumption.[21] Even though sheep infected with scrapie had been slaughtered for human consumption for hundreds of years without any apparent ill effect, it was not clear if cattle infected with BSE would pose the same minimal risk.[22] Based on this concern, the SWP reasoned that the risk of BSE transmission to humans might be similarly "remote," but it could not be ruled out.[23] With cattle, although the affected cattle's heads were removed and discarded, the committee members did not believe that this precaution was a sufficient safeguard against the spread of disease because other parts of the animals might have been infected. They immediately recommended that the entire carcasses of all BSE-affected animals be destroyed by incineration (or a comparable method) and not be allowed for human consumption; the recommendation was accepted and implemented.[24]

At the same time, Rees recommended to John MacGregor, minister of MAFF, that feeding meat and bone meal (MBM) to cattle be banned in order to reduce new infections. MBM is ground-up livestock (the parts not typically eaten by humans, such as the offal—intestines, spleen, and spinal column), which is used as feed. Some of the sheep and cattle parts in MBM could have been contaminated with BSE prions. MBM had been included in cattle feed for decades because of its high protein content, as a way of increasing milk production. Rees recommended that the ban be voluntary, but if the feed industry did not comply, then it could be made mandatory under the Animal Health Act of 1981. The ban would not apply to chickens and pigs because they did not appear susceptible to the disease, and—as most MBM was fed to these animals anyway—he predicted the economic impact would not be significant.[25]

In June 1988, Keith Meldrum replaced Rees as chief veterinary officer for MAFF, and his first act was to explain to the feed industry that there was strong evidence linking BSE with the use of MBM in animal feed. He said that the ban would not apply to animals other than cattle and that exports would continue.[26]

Although the industry pleaded for a two-month grace period to clear its stocks of animal feed, the MAFF minister refused on the grounds of the risk of further spread of the disease by pandering to industry wishes. The Bovine Spongiform Encephalopathy Order was signed on June 14, 1988, and went into full effect one week later.[27]

Before its second meeting in November 1988, the SWP members increased their knowledge about spongiform encephalopathies by reading the scientific literature, communicating with colleagues, and reviewing information provided by MAFF.[28] During this time, the SWP was also informed that experiments on mice injected with BSE-infected bovine brain matter were showing signs of disease 290 days postinoculation, providing evidence that BSE was transmissible.[29]

The epidemiologic studies begun in June 1987 by Wilesmith were showing signs typical of food-borne outbreaks: the data pointed to a common source exposure over an extended period of time. The vast majority of the cases were in young female dairy cattle in the southern counties of England. Cattle in Scotland had the lowest risk for getting BSE. Wilesmith and his colleagues hypothesized that the affected cattle were exposed to a transmissible agent in the cattle feed, likely MBM, and that they were exposed beginning in winter 1981–82.[30]

In the early 1980s, changes had occurred in MBM production that might have contributed to the development of BSE. An increase in the sheep population from 22 to 35 million, with a concomitant increase in the number of cases of scrapie, led to more infected sheep carcasses being taken to rendering plants that produced MBM. Also, whole sheep heads were sent for rendering instead of skinning them and removing the brains, as had been the previous practice.[31]

Another change within the rendering industry was also considered a potential contributor to the BSE outbreak. "Batch processing" in small rendering facilities had been largely replaced by high-volume "continuous rendering" in large plants. Those large rendering facilities used lower temperatures than those used for batch processing. The higher temperatures might have inactivated the prions. They also stopped using hydrocarbon solvents and terminal heat treatments for fat extraction because of two developments: since the mid- to late-1970s, the lowered value of extracted fat (tallow) made it no longer economically prudent to continue the practice,[32] and several industrial accidents had occurred when the solvent exploded.[33] These changes might have inadvertently promoted the transmission of dangerous prions. Of note, two rendering plants in Scotland, where there were fewer cases of BSE, continued to use the solvent extraction process.[34] Any of these factors could have allowed increased levels of contaminated material to enter the cattle feed and increased the risk of disease transmission.

At its November 1988 meeting, the SWP recommended that the 1998 Bovine Spongiform Encephalopathy Order—which had been set to expire at the end of the year—remain in effect indefinitely. In addition, milk from BSE-infected cows should be destroyed, and the offspring of affected cattle should be monitored.[35]

The SWP met two more times, in December 1988 and February 1989, before issuing its final report on February 9, 1989, to John MacGregor and Kenneth Clarke, secretary of state for health.[36] The report noted that the practice of feeding animal proteins to herbivores opened up new avenues for disease transmission, but it acknowledged that the rendering industry provided an important service in processing animal waste material for animal feed and industrial purposes. It recommended that the practice should continue if a rendering process capable of destroying all pathogens could be assured.[37]

In its concluding remarks, the SWP noted that its deliberations were limited by the paucity of research, but it believed that the transmission of BSE to humans was unlikely. The SWP warned, however, that if this assessment were wrong, then the outcome could be extremely serious.[38] The committee suggested that if the disease were to appear in humans, it would closely resemble CJD; therefore, surveillance for unusual cases of CJD was warranted. It also recommended that baby food producers avoid the use of ruminant offal and thymus, but that adult food should be labeled so that consumers could make an informed choice.[39]

The report stimulated intense media interest in whether human food was adequately protected against possible contamination from cattle harboring BSE. In June 1989, the MAFF minister announced the plan to ban specified bovine offal (SBO) from all human food and in July of that year, the European Commission banned the United Kingdom from sending live cattle born before July 18, 1988, to other member states. Four months later, the Bovine Offal (Prohibition) Regulations were put into force in England and Wales; equivalent regulations were put into effect two months later in Scotland and Northern Ireland.[40]

In its final report, the SWP also recommended establishing a research advisory committee to address the scientific uncertainties surrounding BSE. Dr. David Tyrrell, a virologist and director of the UK Medical Research

Council Common Cold Unit, chaired this new committee, the Consultative Committee on Research into Spongiform Encephalopathies (known as the Tyrrell Committee). Jointly administered by MAFF and the Department of Health, the five-member committee[41] met three times between March and May 1989 to recommend and prioritize research projects. By June 1989, the committee had completed a report that recommended, among other things, monitoring BSE cases in cattle and surveillance of all cases of CJD for potential human victims of BSE.[42]

Although the Medical Research Council[43] had access to prepublication copies of the final Tyrrell Report, official publication was delayed until January 1990 because of funding concerns. John Gummer, who succeeded MacGregor as minister of MAFF, believed that the government had no other option but to fund the high-priority research projects recommended by the committee—otherwise, the government would be open to criticism. But the ambitious research agenda set forth by the Tyrrell Committee would have to be funded by monies already appropriated by Parliament: the Treasury would not provide additional funds. According to David Maclean, MAFF parliamentary secretary, MAFF was already spending approximately £1.3 million (approximately $2.3 million) in the current fiscal year and was planning on spending an additional £3.9 million over the next three fiscal years on BSE issues. The secretaries of state for health and for education and science would have to allocate additional funds from their respective departments.[44]

The Tyrrell Committee also recommended that a standing expert group be formed to oversee research coordination and cooperation across the disciplines. Dr. Hilary Pickles, principal medical officer with the Department of Health (DH), and Robert Lowson, head of the Animal Division at MAFF, had reservations about such a committee. Pickles thought it would be inappropriate for a group to report to both DH and MAFF; there could be political risks if funding did not match the group's recommendations. Lowson did not want a committee that would produce reports for publication. Nevertheless, in January 1990, Kenneth Clarke and John Gummer approved the establishment of the Spongiform Encephalopathy Advisory Committee (SEAC). This committee, chaired by Tyrrell, would review research and give policy advice but would not produce reports.[45]

In response to the recommendations of both the SWP and Tyrrell committees, Dr. Robert Will, a consultant neurologist at Western General Hospital in Edinburgh and a member of the Tyrrell Committee, began the CJD surveillance project in May 1990. The Department of Health and the Scottish Office Home and Health Department jointly funded the project.[46] The initial reports of spongiform encephalopathy began with classical Creutzfeldt-Jacob cases or those of other known human spongiform encephalopathies.[47]

The fact that some of these CJD cases occurred in cattle farmers gained some attention but their presenting signs and pathology were indistinguishable from those of classical Creutzfeldt-Jakob disease. Each new CJD case with any apparent connection to cattle was reviewed by SEAC. By late 1995, however, a new pattern of spongiform encephalopathy emerged with a cluster of younger cases with unique pathologies and presenting signs different from those of classical CJD. SEAC reviewed the data from the surveillance unit and ultimately concluded in early 1996 that a new type of human spongiform encephalopathy had occurred.[48]

In March 1996, Stephen Dorrell, member of Parliament and Department of Health secretary of state, shared the SEAC assessment with the British Parliament, announcing that 10 people had developed a distinct variant of Creutzfeldt-Jakob disease (vCJD) over the preceding 14 months and that the most likely cause for the disease was exposure to BSE.[49]

By December 2003, a total of 143 people in the UK had been diagnosed as definite (autopsy-verified) or probable variant CJD cases. Their median age was 29, in contrast to the median age of 65 for classical CJD. Furthermore, death generally occurred within 7 to 14 months after the first neurological and psychiatric symptoms developed, a much longer disease progression than typically seen with classical CJD.[50]

In the same time period, the epidemic of BSE in British cows continued to grow in massive numbers. From 1987 to 2003, more than 180,000 British cows were confirmed to have BSE. The epidemic peaked in 1992 but declined after measures such as the elimination of offal from cattle entering the feed chain were adopted to prevent further spread.[51]

Laboratory studies, which had been recommended by SWP and SEAC, provided further scientific evidence that the agent that caused BSE in cows also caused vCJD in humans. Two independent groups of scientists found that BSE could be transmitted to inoculated mice and concluded that the prion that caused BSE also caused variant CJD.[52] As the details of the BSE/vCJD crisis became widely known, the public response was predictable. In April 1996, the editors of *The Lancet,* a prestigious British medical journal, wrote that the BSE episode highlighted the secretive and inadequate way in which government officials obtain expert scientific advice. The ministers appoint expert committees which meet and review the evidence in private. The commissioning department then issues short, bald statements of their conclusions or recommendations. The process could be handled better by using a separate, independent agency that reports to the public, not to the policy makers.[53]

On January 12, 1998, Lord Nicholas Addison Phillips, chief justice of England and Wales, began a public inquiry into the British government's handling of the BSE/vCJD crisis.[54] The Phillips Inquiry documented the failings of the scientific advisory system, including an overreliance on outside experts who were known personally by government officials. The inquiry found fault with SWP committee members for basing conclusions on MAFF epidemiological data even though they had never actually seen the data.[55]

The Phillips Inquiry found that the government had taken reasonable, but not timely, measures. The MAFF and Department of Health leaders, but not the politicians, were to be blamed for the poor handling of the crisis. They did not adequately communicate the risk of acquiring BSE to the public, even though scientific evidence was accumulating that such a risk did exist. The inquiry concluded that the government had deceived the media and the public for a decade by insisting that beef was safe to eat.[56]

Erik Millstone and Patrick van Zwanenberg, researchers in science policy at the University of Sussex, Brighton, disagreed with the conclusions of the Phillips Inquiry. They argued that the report underestimated the extent and severity of the failures of the BSE crisis. According to them, MAFF's primary policy agenda was to assure consumers that British beef was safe to eat. The central issue was one of legitimacy, since public trust could be justified only if policymaking involved both scientific and political legitimacy. They argued that policymaking was not legitimate given the conditions of the BSE crisis in which scientific knowledge was highly uncertain and incomplete.[57]

VIEWS OF THE CRISIS

One of the leaders involved with the BSE crisis was Dr. Keith Meldrum, chief veterinary officer (CVO) of England, Scotland, and Wales from 1988 to 1997. When he was the CVO, he also represented the United Kingdom at the World Organization for Animal Health (OIE) and served on the Standing Veterinary Committee of the European Union (EU). Here is his reflection on his time as CVO:

> BSE was a massive animal health challenge with incredible complexity. It was a totally new disease with a lot of uncertainty surrounding it. Before I became CVO, I had been involved with the recycling of animal proteins and the use of animal feeds. Nobody ever suggested that scrapie might affect cattle.
>
> My primary responsibility as CVO was to advise ministers. I was also responsible for executive decisions such as confirming the existence of an outbreak and for all sorts of negotiations in Brussels and elsewhere. By law, the CVO is responsible for the confirmation of the existence of a notifiable disease. The minister was responsible for the strategic decisions such as banning MBM for use in feed for ruminants. The minister would make such decisions based on advice from the CVO and from others such

as advisory committees. The minister had to make the ultimate decision because he was answerable to the House of Commons and would have to defend it. Ministers invariably would accept the CVO's advice. I had no problems working with them. It is important to note that they wouldn't just take my advice, but they would also take advice from people in advisory committees.

BSE was an unknown disease, and very little was known about CJD. There were only 30 to 50 or so cases of CJD per year in the UK before vCJD was diagnosed in 1996. Very few people had seen it. After Southwood [the Southwood committee], there was the SEAC [Spongiform Encephalopathy Advisory Committee]. It was helpful to have a standing advisory committee. As CVO, I would review the opinions of these committees.

However, there is a danger in being surrounded by all sorts of advisory committees, and it is important to know how the members of the advisory committees are appointed. You must look at their recommendations carefully. Is the advice based on scientific evidence or on opinion?

For example, Sir John Pattison,[58] who was the chair of the SEAC committee, went public and said that there could be half a million cases of vCJD. It was a massive overestimate—a pure figure off the wall. It was totally unhelpful and frightened people to death. There was no scientific evidence to support that statement.

Many of the decisions that were made during the BSE crisis were inspirational. They were sound then, and they haven't been changed in any significant way since. For example, the SBO ban of 1989 is still in place even though members of the opposition party in Parliament criticized it. They didn't change it when they took over following the general election in 1997. The decision to ban MBM was based on sound epidemiological science done by John Wilesmith. His work was spot on.

I think the ban on SBO offals was inspirational. Southwood had recommended that cattle with BSE should be destroyed and that some bovine offals should not be put in baby food. We weren't sure why they focused on just baby food, but we took that recommendation and considered whether there should be a wider restriction on the use of bovine material in human food. On the basis of a risk assessment, we concluded that certain bovine materials, including brain and spinal cord, thymus, spleen, and some intestines of healthy cattle, except calves, should not be permitted to be used in any human food. This was a good decision. We took out of the food chain a massive load of potentially infectious material.

However, a better job could have been done enforcing the SBO ban to ensure that it was properly implemented in slaughterhouses and that all spinal cord was removed and destroyed. Local authorities were responsible for meat hygiene and inspection until the Meat Hygiene Service was formed in 1995. It was hard to get uniformity across the country to remove brains and spinal cords from sub-clinically affected cattle [cattle that had BSE but were not yet showing signs of illness] in the slaughterhouses.

We were responsible for animal health and the Department of Health was responsible for human health. Too often, I got sucked into commenting on food safety at press briefings and in interviews. If the CMO [chief medical officer] didn't want to answer these questions, we shouldn't have either. This was a lesson that I learned the hard way. Advice regarding food safety relevant to BSE should have come from the Department of Health.

Ministers had ultimate responsibility, but at the end of the day, the buck stopped with me. There was a massive inquiry into BSE led by Lord Phillips. The CVO was in the firing line while ministers got away with it. My advice for future CVOs: be very careful and protect yourself to ensure that you cannot become the scapegoat.

I would insist on direct access to the secretary of state [the most senior minister] at all times, in the way that I did. The ministers must support every important decision, and their agreement must be recorded. I would recommend that all CVOs keep a diary of all major meetings, events, and decisions taken. The buck stops with the CVO, and the CVO should stand up for his/her beliefs and principles.

The report of the inquiry into BSE took up 16 volumes. It showed how much effort we put into BSE.[59]

The BSE crisis was unique in that it spanned a decade from the first identified cows to the first identified human victims. Five different members of Parliament served as ministers of agriculture during those 10 years. John MacGregor was the first of those ministers. He became minister of MAFF in 1987 just as the BSE crisis began to unfold and served in that office until 1989. Here is his view of the crisis:

As minister, I had overall responsibility and the leading role during the period from 1988 to 1989 when BSE first appeared as a crisis. The knowledge that BSE could be transmitted to humans came seven years after my time. It was an unknown disease. For many months in 1987–88, our problem was that we didn't know what it was and what caused it. We needed clarity from the scientists.

We assembled the Southwood Committee in order to bring in the leading experts for the best science advice possible. . . . Southwood first recommended banning ruminant offals from baby food. I felt that if the scientists recommended that there was a danger in baby food, I thought, "What about all foods?" On reflection, I decided to go further than just baby food. Professor Southwood felt that the priority and the scientific necessity were for baby food but was happy to go along with my view.

As an MP, I was spending a lot of my time with my constituents, which for many years were in a farming area, so I was familiar with agriculture issues before I became a minister. But I don't have a background in science, so I relied on the scientists, including the chief veterinary officer [CVO], for advice in areas such as BSE. The CVO reported to me.

Outbreaks require very fast responses. The media will be fast to report on any food scare, so it is best to be open with them. Unfortunately, BSE was not easy to understand. The moment cattle began to fall about in the fields, we were trying to understand what it was. The delay was frustrating for me but I believe, as did the Phillips Inquiry, that we took all the right measures. After my time as minister, the implementation of the [MBM] feed ban policy was not fully enforced. Some material still got from the rendering facilities to farms, and monitoring was not 100 percent. That could have been done better.

Since that time, an independent body, the Food Standards Agency [FSA][60] was set up. The FSA has a separate board and chair. I always thought it to be essential that the chair should be a good scientist who is able to communicate to the general public, and I believe that was achieved. The FSA establishes food safety and standards. It is now the one to handle food crises, which has shifted some of the responsibility, but it's still the ministers who make the policy decisions.[61]

CONCLUSION

The main mission of MAFF, like most departments of agriculture, was to promote agriculture even as it regulated the agricultural industry. The arrangement creates a potential conflict of interest between the needs of the industry and of consumers.[62] The Phillips Inquiry did not see this arrangement as problematic, however, and instead considered it an advantage because it combined everything under one minister.[63]

Lord MacGregor's narrative suggests that the Southwood advisory committee sought to avoid placing undue hardship on the agricultural industry. The minister took its advice and applied his own common sense by banning potentially dangerous materials from all human food—rather than limiting the ban to baby food. In contrast, Gummer, the subsequent minister of MAFF, decided not to ban mechanically recovered meat and was subsequently criticized by the press for trying to show that meat was safe by forcing his daughter to eat a hamburger.

MAFF leaders confronted a difficult crisis in which little was known about the disease, its cause, or its transmission. Although it was unknown for years that humans could be infected by eating contaminated meat, the initial assumption that BSE would behave like scrapie was optimistic but, unfortunately, wrong. The Phillips Inquiry criticized the leaders for misleading the public.

Millstone and Zwanenberg recommended several ways that countries could improve scientific and political legitimacy in crisis decision making. They suggested that in order to reduce the risk of political influence, expert scientific advisory groups should deliberate separately from the agencies that seek their advice. Furthermore, scientific discussions should be open to the public and the questions they consider should address specific policy objectives—using all available evidence to assess potential risks. Most important, uncertainties need to be identified and acknowledged by scientists and policymakers.[64] There is a risk, however, in opening all preliminary scientific deliberations to the public: many reporters and laypeople do not understand the complexities involved and might misinterpret speculation as fact.

Parliament responded to the BSE crisis by restructuring the government. As Lord MacGregor mentioned, the Food Standards Agency was created to be an independent body that eliminated the potential conflict of interest raised by having one agency both promote and regulate an industry. In the end, however, the elected officials would remain responsible for policy decisions.

One of the findings in the BSE inquiry was that the CVO did not have the degree of independence afforded to the chief medical officer (CMO). Unlike the CMO, the CVO did not have the authority to state his or her opinions publicly or give advice to the public. The CVO position in MAFF was not a parallel position with the CMO in the health department. The CVO ranked at the level of deputy CMO, possibly hindering cross-disciplinary communication and collaboration between the two professional leaders.

According to Sir Donald Acheson (CMO during the first six years of the crisis), however, the CMO and CVO did work together.[65] The CVO role was expanded after Lord Phillips of Worth Matravers recommended in the BSE Inquiry Report that the CVO should, like the CMO, be able to give independent advice to the public.[66]

The relationship between the CVO and the minister was clear: the CVO advised the minister in charge. There was no evidence of role confusion between the elected official and the bureaucratic professional. This clarity of roles might stem from the fact that veterinarians typically do not give health advice to people, so the public might not expect them to play a major leadership role in a crisis that could affect the public's health.

The BSE epidemic was a complicated crisis that spanned a decade and involved many leaders. Before scientific information about the new disease accumulated, leaders had to make decisions based on best advice and common sense while taking into account industry and consumer concerns. Because of the disease's novelty and slow course, scientific understanding took years to develop, hindering policy decisions and actions to prevent further spread to animals and humans. MAFF officials initially responded to the outbreak by downplaying the problem in order to prevent public panic and unnecessary harm to the agricultural industry. Although this approach to risk communication is understandable and widespread, the bureaucratic tendency to keep secrets[67] in the long run erodes public trust and is counterproductive in promoting public health.

Unfortunately, British exports of cattle during the 1980s and early 1990s may have contributed to cases of vCJD in the importing countries, including France, Italy, Ireland, the Netherlands, Spain, and Portugal. France, Ireland, and the Netherlands received the largest number of these exports, and they have had the highest number of cases of vCJD outside of the UK. By September 2006, a total of 196 cases of vCJD had been reported globally, but 82 percent (162) occurred in the UK. Some of the international victims might have been exposed while they were living in the UK, but many cases occurred in those who never visited the country. In other words, some of those cases probably came from exposure to indigenous bovine products. In 2000, many continental European countries banned specified bovine offal in the human food supply in an effort to minimize human exposure to BSE. Sadly, those exposed before the bans were implemented could develop vCJD.[68]

THE VITAL LINK BETWEEN
ANIMAL AND HUMAN HEALTH

Part II

THE FOOT-AND-MOUTH DISEASE CRISIS

Five years after the first human cases of BSE were announced to Parliament, the British agricultural industry was hit with another devastating blow: an outbreak of foot-and-mouth disease (FMD).

FMD primarily affects livestock: cows, goats, pigs, and sheep. Pregnant animals typically abort their fetuses, and young animals may die. Milk production can be permanently impaired, and infected animals can develop permanent deformities.[1] The virus that causes FMD produces fever, loss of appetite, blisters in the mouth and on the foot, teats, and udder; and inflammation of the females' mammary glands. The incubation period (the length of time from infection to the appearance of illness) ranges from 2 to 14 days. Animals can be contagious before they show signs of illness.

Pigs are frequently the first species to become sick with FMD, often after eating infected garbage;[2] they generate large numbers of virions (virus particles) that spread to other animals.[3] The disease is hard to diagnose in sheep because the lesions are less pronounced; however, because they produce fewer virions, they can spread the disease widely without detection. Cattle, on the other hand, show severe signs of the disease and suffer considerably.

The virus spreads quickly and over great distances with ease: it can spread by air up to 60 kilometers (about 37 miles) overland and 300 kilometers (about 186 miles) across the open ocean. Humans can inadvertently spread the virus on their clothes or shoes; vehicles and inanimate objects also can carry it. The virus mutates readily during replication, leading to new strains. O pan-Asian is the most virulent strain of FMD.[4]

Scientific evidence suggests that the O pan-Asian strain emerged in India as early as 1982.[5] In the 1990s, it spread across the Middle East to Europe and across Asia to the Far East. In 2000, it jumped to South Africa.[6]

Severe FMD outbreaks occurred in the UK in 1922, 1924, 1954, and 1967. Each led to government inquiries that emphasized the dangers of feeding pigs untreated garbage, the importance of tagging animals to aid in identification, the necessity of speed for outbreak containment, the impact of animal movements on disease spread, and the critical role of the availability of large numbers of veterinarians.[7]

During the 1967 FMD crisis, the military was recruited to help slaughter and dispose of almost 500,000 animal carcasses. A subsequent inquiry, the *Northumberland Report*,[8] recommended that a permanent liaison between the Ministry of Agriculture and the military be established to help in the slaughter and disposal of animal carcasses in future crises.[9]

The 1967 crisis affected *primarily* cattle and pigs—not sheep—and cost the country around 150 million pounds (approximately $413 million in 1967 dollars). The outbreak lasted more than seven months and required the slaughter of 434,000 cattle, pigs, and sheep before it could be stamped out.[10]

After the 1967 FMD crisis, many changes occurred in agriculture in the United Kingdom. The practice of livestock farming became increasingly fragmented and regionalized; farmers kept livestock scattered in far-flung landholdings in the north and west of the country. The population of sheep, which serves as a silent transmission vector for FMD, increased by almost 60 percent, and farmers moved their sheep around the country to take advantage of regional climate changes and grass growth patterns. The European Union (EU) Common Agriculture Policy required that farmers have all their sheep available for annual inspection during the months of February and March, so the movement of millions of sheep would occur during that time.

UK government oversight of livestock changed; the ranks of the State Veterinary Service were reduced by two-thirds. Livestock inspections were outsourced to private-practice veterinarians. The number of veterinarians practicing large animal (livestock) medicine decreased with time. Yet, the public's concern about animal welfare increased.[11]

The last outbreak of FMD in the UK before the one in 2001 occurred in 1981 on the Isle of Wight. The outbreak began after the virus traveled 241 kilometers (150 miles) across the open waters of the English Channel from Brittany.[12] It was a relatively minor outbreak in a single dairy herd. It was most notable for the distance the virus traveled from Brittany. The UK was free of FMD for the next twenty years, and the lessons learned from the previous FMD crises were forgotten.

On the morning of February 19, 2001, Craig Kirby, the resident veterinarian at Cheale's Abattoir (a slaughterhouse) in Essex, England, conducted a routine veterinary inspection and found distressed pigs waiting to be slaughtered. He noticed that the pigs had mouth blisters that were due to either swine vesicular disease (a minor viral disease of pigs), or FMD. These two diseases are indistinguishable in pigs without confirmation by a laboratory test.[13]

Kirby called the local State Veterinary Service office in Chelmsford to report his findings. Two Ministry of Agriculture, Fisheries and Food (MAFF) veterinarians came to the abattoir and agreed with Kirby's concerns. They took blood and tissue samples from the infected animals and drove the specimens 70 miles to the Pirbright Laboratory at the Institute for Animal Health in Surrey. Unfortunately, no one at the laboratory was aware that the samples were coming, so they sat overnight at the laboratory before being analyzed.[14]

The veterinarians restricted movement of all livestock in and near the abattoir and advised farmers within a five-mile zone to check their livestock for symptoms of the disease.[15]

By the next morning, February 20, some of the infected pigs became extremely distressed, so they were killed to end their suffering. No further actions were taken until later in the day when the laboratory confirmed FMD in the specimens. Dr. Alex Donaldson, head of the Pirbright Laboratory, came to the abattoir in the evening to confirm the clinical evidence of FMD in the pigs and shortly thereafter the pigs began to be slaughtered. The operation continued until the early hours of the next morning.

By then, however, animals at the farm adjacent to the abattoir had become infected and had to be slaughtered. Three other FMD outbreaks simultaneously occurred around the country, and the export of livestock and animal products was quickly banned. Three days later, animal movement was restricted to decrease the risk of further disease spread. The government ordered that all livestock markets and abattoirs be shut down as the slaughter of animals began.[16]

Life in the countryside rapidly and dramatically changed. The owners of infected farms and their neighbors were quarantined in their homes. All deliveries to farms stopped, including the delivery of letters. All recreation in rural areas ceased, as people were not allowed to take walks or go outside. Tourism was discouraged. Even dogs could not go out in the fields, and horses had to stay in their stalls.[17]

On February 24, MAFF veterinarians identified Burnside farm in Heddon-on-the-Wall, Northumberland, as the possible source of the outbreak.[18] Large numbers of farmers sent sows (female pigs) that were too old for breeding to this farm. The Northumberland farm owners typically kept the pigs for two to five days and then transported them to Cheale's Abattoir where the first cases were identified.[19]

Two brothers, Bobby and Ronnie Waugh, owned the Burnside farm. The brothers denied noticing anything wrong with their pigs in the preceding weeks. But an anonymous complaint in December had stated that the pigs were living in squalor and were in poor condition, leading to a visit by a MAFF state veterinarian on December 22, 2000, who found the animals at that time to be healthy. An animal welfare group said, however, that the farm had been tipped off about the complaint and inspection. The group stated that the pigs were living in the midst of rotting animal carcasses and were eating garbage and baby piglets. Nonetheless, a subsequent annual routine MAFF inspection on January 25, 2001, had given the farm a clean bill of health.[20]

MAFF officials subsequently determined that Ronnie Waugh fed his pigs garbage (i.e., swill) from food waste instead of formulated feed to save money. Alan and Kenneth Clement, the swill suppliers, collected garbage from restaurants, schools, and cafes and took it to the farm where it lay untreated.[21] Boiling swill at 93.3°C (200°F) for four hours is required to inactivate viruses. Officials were also investigating as a possible source of the outbreak meat smuggled from Asia by an importer who was avoiding dock and airport inspection fees. The smuggled meat was found concealed inside a shipment of household goods and had been labeled for a Chinese restaurant.[22]

On February 25, cattle on a farm in Highhampton, Devon, 400 miles from the Burnside farm, tested positive for FMD. The farm had 1,500 sheep and the owner, William Cleave, also had livestock scattered across 10 other farms in Devon and two in Cornwall.[23] MAFF veterinarians determined that 18 sheep worth less than £900 ($1,296) were likely responsible for the spread of the virus. Cleave had purchased the sheep from Hexham market in Northumberland. The sheep had originally come from Prestwick Hall Farm, Ponteland, in Northumberland, which was located five kilometers (three miles) northeast of the Burnside farm. Wind probably spread the virus from the pigs to the sheep.[24]

Six days before the government identified FMD in the country, the sheep had been taken from Prestwick Hall Farm to Hexham market to be sold along with 3,800 other sheep and 85 cattle that belonged to about 120 other farmers. The sheep were likely incubating the disease and were therefore infectious. Some of the sheep went to a butcher; others went to a farm in Lancashire. A dealer bought the rest and took them to Longtown market in Cumbria.

At least 24,500 sheep passed through the markets over a 10-day period and were potentially exposed. By the time the first pig was identified at the abattoir, nearly 57 farms in 16 counties had been infected. Some sheep had been exported to France.[25]

Farmers were demanding more protections for livestock, and they blamed a number of factors for contributing to the development and spread of FMD. They wanted more inspections at ports of foreign meat products that could bring in disease. They demanded that the public not be allowed to bring in cooked meat from abroad. They were concerned about the dramatic decline in the number of abattoirs from 1,000 to 340 over a 10-year period. They believed that the shortage of abattoirs meant that they had to transport their livestock greater distances to be slaughtered, thus increasing the risk of infection with the disease. Abattoir owners complained that they could not afford to deal with the EU bureaucracy and inspection fees. Nick Brown, the minister of MAFF, sent a letter to his cabinet colleagues asking for suggestions on how to improve the situation.[26]

Meanwhile, farmers in France were worried. The last major French outbreak of FMD had occurred 25 years previously and had been economically devastating. Farmers contemplated slaughtering all the animals that had been imported from Great Britain during the previous few months, and in the end, they decided to kill 30,000 sheep as a precaution.[27]

Worse yet, the scientists at the Pirbright Laboratory identified the FMD virus as the virulent O pan-Asian strain. Paul Kitching, the head of the Department of Exotic Diseases at the laboratory, said in a *London Times* interview that the pan-Asian strain usually caused outbreaks in developing countries. He was shocked that an outbreak with this viral strain was occurring in the UK.[28]

On March 6, Jim Scudamore, the UK chief veterinarian officer (CVO) announced that he was optimistic that the FMD crisis would be quickly brought under control. He said that almost every case had been convincingly traced to the first outbreak at the Burnside farm in Heddon-on-the-Wall, but it would not be possible to declare the crisis over until at least 30 days had passed without new cases developing. By then, 40,000 animals had been slaughtered.[29]

Sir John Krebs, chairman of the Food Standards Agency, sought out experts in mathematical modeling to help with the crisis. He hosted an ad hoc group of experts to discuss what information they needed from MAFF to predict the course of the epidemic. Four different teams began working on the problem.[30]

By March 10, a second viral wave developed with 127 new cases confirmed.[31] Nick Brown, the minister of MAFF, repeatedly assured the public that the FMD crisis was under control. As more FMD cases appeared, the press became increasingly skeptical of the government's assurances. Every week, the number of infected farms appeared to be doubling.[32]

By March 12, a team of mathematical modelers at the Veterinary Laboratories Agency predicted that FMD might balloon to 1,000 to 2,000 cases from the current 182 cases. In Scotland, FMD outbreaks were exploding in its southwest region, Dumfries and Galloway. The Scottish Executive[33] and the National Farmer's Union of Scotland developed a plan to save the valuable cattle populations in the north. They decided to create firewalls by slaughtering all sheep within a 3-kilometer (1.86-mile) radius of a confirmed infected farm. The Scottish Executive subsequently met with Prime Minister Tony Blair at Downing Street for high-level meetings to coordinate English-Scottish disease control efforts.[34]

A March 14 editorial in the *London Times* stated:

> The comfort to be gained from Nick Brown's assurances that foot-and-mouth disease is "under control" diminishes with each new case. It is growing exponentially with more than 200 outbreaks and has spread to France.[35]

On March 15, Blair announced that there would be a massive cull of animals throughout the UK. More than one million sheep and tens of thousands of healthy cattle and pigs would be slaughtered in an attempt to contain FMD. Nick Brown announced the UK's five key disease control goals: (1) keep uninfected areas of the country free from FMD, (2) halt disease spread in Devon, (3) halt disease spread in the north of England and southwest Scotland, (4) eliminate infection in sheep that passed through dealers known to have handled infected sheep, and (5) minimize disease spread from the Longtown, Northampton, and Welshpool markets.[36]

The next day, a mathematical modeling team at Imperial College, London, advised MAFF that reducing the delay between diseased animal identification and slaughter would be critical for disease containment. The team hoped that the policy of the 3-kilometer (1.86-mile) cull announced on March 15 would help contain the spreading epidemic.

Unfortunately, the implementation of the preemptive cull policy would not begin until March 22 in Scotland and March 28 in the UK.

As farmers remained isolated in their homes, they became increasingly depressed and some turned suicidal. Brian Oakley, a 54-year-old farmer of a 26 acre sheep farm near Oswestry, hanged himself a week after FMD was first discovered. A close friend said Oakley could not cope with the restrictions and was worried about his sheep.[37]

The Prince of Wales donated £500,000 ($720,000) to help the farmers cope with the ongoing crisis. He held private talks with Nick Brown at St. James's Palace. The gift prompted the press to speculate that the prince thought the government was not doing enough to help the farmers cope with the psychological stress and impending financial ruin. Some insurance companies stopped selling FMD-protection policies, and others notified farmers living near infected areas that they would not be able to renew their policies until further notice.[38]

On March 19, Scudamore announced that an extended slaughter of more than 300,000 sheep would begin shortly in northern Cumbria in an attempt to halve the spread of FMD. He was booed when he arrived at a livestock market near Carlisle, the largest city in Cumbria, for talks with private veterinary surgeons and leaders of the National Farmer's Union to explain the rationale for the extensive cull. By that time, one month had passed since the crisis began and more than 300,000 animals had been slaughtered.[39]

Upon his arrival, farmers presented Scudamore with documents outlining the bureaucratic mistakes made in handling the crisis. The documents showed that MAFF had a shortage of veterinarians, delayed valuing livestock before slaughter, and delayed slaughter and disposal of infected carcasses. One farmer complained that carcasses remained on his farm for four days, and the smell was "diabolical." Another farmer complained that it took five days for his herd to be slaughtered, giving the virus time to spread to other farms.[40]

With no end in sight, farmers in Cumbria began rioting and demanded that the CVO dispose of infected livestock more quickly and stop the slaughter of uninfected animals. One farmer threatened to kill a MAFF official, so the police confiscated his shotgun. Farmers demanded that the army be brought in to assist. The Prince of Wales's Own Regiment at Preston sent 150 soldiers to Cumbria to help remove infected animal carcasses.[41]

On March 21, the ad hoc group of mathematical modelers met again at the Food Standards Agency and concluded that FMD was out of control. The group members predicted that the outbreak might not peak until early May. The group met regularly for the next six months.[42]

The next day, Prime Minister Tony Blair held emergency meetings with Nick Brown to discuss the situation and, on March 26, Blair took charge of the FMD crisis.[43] He began chairing daily meetings in Cabinet Office Briefing Room A (known as the "COBRA" war room) located in the Cabinet Office basement and connected to 10 Downing Street. The room, reserved for national emergencies, became the crisis management center. Maps showing the spread of the epidemic, rural pathways, national parks, and tourist sites were hung on the walls. Officials staffed the room from early morning to late at night with regular updates for the prime minister. Details included veterinarian availability, army personnel, vaccine availability, and statistics on the scale of FMD spread.[44] After Blair took command of the outbreak response, the number of infected animals awaiting slaughter rose by 73 percent.[45]

A small team of military officers began to work at MAFF. Nick Brown reportedly snapped, "This is still a civilian ministry. We are not under military control yet." Nevertheless, the Ministry of Defense took an increasingly larger role in the crisis. Jim Scudamore would be in charge of strategy with the assistance of two deputies, and army logistics officers and veterinarians would coordinate the day-to-day control of the outbreak. The FMD outbreak, preceded by the decade-long BSE crisis, led to growing calls for the decommissioning and replacement of MAFF.[46]

The shortage of veterinarians became critical. Once a veterinarian entered an infected farm, he or she was classified as "dirty" and could not work at another farm until a specified period of time had passed. This meant that the number of veterinarians needed to work on infected farms increased dramatically as the number of these farms grew. Brown appealed to veterinarians worldwide to come to the UK to help with the crisis.[47]

William Hague, a conservative member of Parliament for Richmond, Yorkshire, and leader of the opposition party, wanted complete control of the FMD response to be handed over to the army because MAFF was "hopelessly overstretched." The army had, by then, taken over the task of burying and reburying animal carcasses. In Durham, almost 900 animals had to be reburied because of concerns that they would pollute an underground spring. MAFF and Department of the Environment officials became embroiled in arguments over burial sites, animal movements, and EU regulations. More than a million animals had been killed or targeted for slaughter. It was twice the number of animals slaughtered during the 1967 FMD crisis. A *London Times* editorial characterized the government's response to the crisis as having no leadership or direction.[48]

The mathematical modelers were asked if the epidemic could be brought under control with a cull policy between 1 (0.62 miles) and 1.5 kilometers (0.93 miles) rather than the 3 kilometers (1.86 miles) initially stipulated. If so, then the epidemic might be brought under control with the slaughter of fewer animals. From this initial idea, the policy of the "contiguous cull" emerged. Models suggested that the slaughter of infected animals within 24 hours and preemptive slaughter of healthy animals on contiguous premises within 48 hours might contain the out-of-control epidemic while minimizing the number of animals killed.[49]

Relations between the government and farmers deteriorated further. MAFF officials accused some farmers of submitting fraudulent compensation claims and of illegally moving their livestock. Nick Brown released a report that MAFF had 309 investigations or prosecutions of farmers illegally moving livestock, inadequately disinfecting farm vehicles, and other offences since the beginning of the crisis. MAFF officials blamed farmers for a series of outbreaks in previously unaffected areas.

The army joined the uproar. Major Lucy Giles, a member of the army FMD operation, said they were working with the local police in investigating at least one farmer who intentionally infected his livestock in order to get compensation. A local police spokesperson would not confirm the army's allegations but said that he had heard rumors about the matter. The National Farmers' Union issued a furious reply that farmers were being unfairly blamed for the crisis.[50]

On April 18, a group of veterinarians from Devon sent a letter to MAFF denouncing the contiguous cull policy of needlessly slaughtering thousands of healthy cattle on farms neighboring those with infected herds. Instead, they wanted to save the cattle by keeping them in barns and culling the sheep. They warned that Devon was on the verge of a civil war over the government's handling of the FMD crisis.[51]

On April 21, Dr. Paul Kitching, of the Pirbright Laboratory, announced on television news that the mathematical models used to contain the spread of the disease had been based on 1967 outbreak parameters and they did not apply to the 2001 crisis. MAFF's contiguous cull slaughter policy had been based on faulty advice. A comment in the *London Times* concluded:

> The research, it seems, was wrong, the science was outdated, the slaughter unnecessary, the policy unethical, and the strategy ineffective.[52]

On the night of April 25, a Downing Street spokeswoman announced that the contiguous cull policy was going to be abandoned. The change in policy was precipitated by a calf that was found under a pile of slaughtered animals. Intense media attention on the calf's fate led to public demand that it be allowed to live. The calf's case coincided with a decrease in new FMD cases.[53]

The crisis continued through the spring, summer, and beginning of fall, however, and spread to France, the Netherlands, and the Republic of Ireland. On September 30, the last confirmed case of FMD occurred in Appleby, Cumbria—221 days after the first identified case. On January 22, 2002, the World Organization for Animal Health (known as the OIE, for L'Organisation Mondiale de la Sante Animale, which is based in Paris, France) declared the United Kingdom FMD free and, two weeks later, lifted all export restrictions.

More than 4 million animals had been slaughtered: 3,428,000 sheep, 592,000 cattle, 140,000 pigs, 2,500 goats, and approximately 1,000 deer. An additional 2 million sheep, cattle, and pigs had been slaughtered because movement restrictions prohibited grazing or the animals were no longer marketable.[54]

The economic consequences were enormous. The estimated losses to the UK's gross domestic product were £2 billion ($2.9 billion). The British government gave approximately £1.34 billion ($1.9 billion) to farmers as compensation for their lost livestock. Additional agricultural losses, including export losses, were around £355 million ($511 million). Auction markets, food processors, and slaughterhouses lost an estimated £170 million ($245 million). The tourism industry lost between £1.8 and £2.2 million ($2.6 to 3.2 million).[55]

Not only did animals suffer; human suffering also was profound.[56] Many farmers and their families, made near-prisoners in their homes, felt isolated and abandoned. Children could not go to school. Farmers' psychological trauma correlated with the degree of animal culling and movement restrictions.[57]

At least 3 farmers were confirmed as having committed suicide; however, there were reports that as many as 60 farmers did so.[58] For some, the psychological effects were long lasting. A number of farmers experienced flashbacks analogous to those reported by people suffering from post-traumatic stress disorder.[59]

VIEWS OF THE CRISIS

Dr. Paul Kitching, a veterinarian and researcher, was head of the World Reference Laboratory for FMD at the Institute for Animal Health during the FMD crisis. The Food and Agriculture Organization (FAO) and the OIE designated the Pirbright Laboratory as the World Reference Laboratory for foot-and-mouth disease. In a telephone interview, Kitching noted the following:

> I was responsible for all diagnostics during the foot-and-mouth outbreak. My staff provided diagnostic backup for MAFF in the eradication program. When the initial test came back positive, I notified my boss, Alex Donaldson, who was head of the whole Pirbright site. He called the CVO to give him the results.
>
> The Pirbright Laboratory is not part of MAFF. It is part of the Biotechnology and Biological Sciences Research Council. MAFF didn't have the laboratory capability to handle [biosafety] level-three exotic diseases. We have expertise with a large research staff. I spent the last 20 years of my career going around the world investigating FMD outbreaks and advising how to control FMD. As the designated World Reference Laboratory for the FAO and OIE, we would receive samples from all over the world for diagnosis and advice on suitable vaccine strains.
>
> The FMD virus is always changing, just like the influenza virus. Since there are seven different virus serotypes plus multiple strains within each

serotype, there is no single vaccine against FMD. You have to match the vaccine to the virus. The main problem with the vaccine is that it doesn't prevent infection. It only stops clinical signs, and the animal can still harbor the virus.

When FMD spread from the UK to the Netherlands, the Dutch vaccinated 200,000 animals and then slaughtered them all anyway. They did this because the OIE has trade guidelines that a country must wait six months after vaccination for FMD before it can export again. A country has to wait only three months if the animals are slaughtered. There must be a good reason to vaccinate. It's useful in South American countries where the disease is endemic, but most countries want to avoid FMD becoming endemic.

During the crisis, I had direct contact with the agriculture minister. Other than the prime minister, he was ultimately responsible for eliminating FMD from the country. I had a meeting with the prime minister and advised him not to vaccinate. We didn't know the extent of the outbreak, and it was not possible to completely prevent the movement of animals and virus-contaminated people.

It is normal after winter for farmers to move cattle onto sheep pastures. For example, in Cumbria, farmers were moving cattle out of sheds and onto pastures where sheep were kept. MAFF made it clear that if they used vaccine to protect the cattle, the animals would later be slaughtered.

The disease was probably in the country for three weeks before it was detected. Five hundred adult pigs were infected on one farm. They were eating food waste that wasn't properly cooked. Some of the pigs lost the horns from their toes and couldn't walk. The pigs were sent to a slaughterhouse where they transmitted the disease. Pigs secrete more aerosol virus than do cattle and sheep. If the virus had been the same virus as the 1967–68 virus, it could have spread to the north of Germany and Denmark. In reality, the 2001 outbreak virus didn't spread like that. It spread mostly by illegal movements of infected animals. A lot of this was going on, but it was mostly unintentional. At the end of the epidemic, police were on the roads to check for illegal movements.

The disease was in sheep. Diagnosing FMD in sheep is extremely difficult, and many vets had never seen the disease. I have been diagnosing FMD for 25 to 30 years, and I still have trouble with sheep. You need laboratory support to make a diagnosis, but vets were forced to make slaughter decisions on a large percentage of farms that ultimately tested negative. Massive numbers of animals were needlessly slaughtered.

What was needed was basic disease control. Nothing special. People were not taking adequate precautions. It wasn't rocket science. What happened was that panic set in, and no one sat down to think the problem through.

The mathematical models didn't take into account that the 2001 outbreak was due to a different strain of the Type O virus than that during the 1967–68 outbreak. They assumed airborne spread, and they didn't understand the disease. The previous Royal Society president got all the mathematical modelers together. They agreed not to say anything to the media. That night, Roy Anderson [professor of infectious diseases epidemiology in the Division of Epidemiology, Public Health and Primary Care at Imperial College, London] got on TV to say that the outbreak was out of control. They then took over from the minister of agriculture and sidelined the CVO.

The Food Standards Agency people knew nothing about FMD but were making policy decisions. They listened to the Royal Society mathematical modelers who advised the chief scientist. The chief scientist had the ear of the prime minister. These mathematical models led to the 24/48 slaughter policy in which infected animals must be slaughtered in 24 hours and the animals on neighboring farms be slaughtered in 48 hours. It was a total travesty.

The chief scientist's Science Committee was like the Mad Hatter's tea party: four groups of modelers arguing with one another. Everyone knew that they didn't know much about FMD. And if we challenged them, they would say that we couldn't understand the issues because we didn't know math. Alex and I would sit on the committee and argue about the merits of their models. They totally ignored us, and we were the two FMD experts. In future outbreaks, I would lock up the predictive modelers.[60]

From 2000 to 2005, including throughout the 2001 FMD crisis, Lord John Richard Krebs was chairman of the British Food Standards Agency. Here is his view of the crisis:

I had an official role and an unofficial role during the crisis. In my official role, I was not responsible for animal health but rather for human health. The role of the Food Standards Agency was to regulate abattoirs. With the impending loss of movement of animals, the veterinarians and meat inspectors who work at the abattoirs would potentially be out of work.

In my unofficial role, I was listening to the MAFF officials, Jim Scudamore and Nick Brown going on radio and TV in mid-February telling people that the outbreak was under control. I wondered about that and was concerned that the movement of sheep might have spread the disease farther than they realized. I called some colleagues of mine together, all top experts in modeling, and asked them to come into my office in early March. I invited MAFF officials, but they told me that they were too busy to attend. My colleagues and I met, and they agreed with me that the disease could be spreading more rapidly than thought, but we needed data, including the spatial location of the farms, to test the hypothesis.

I called Brian Bender, the permanent secretary of MAFF, and although he was initially reluctant to provide data, he eventually advised the chief veterinary officer to release the relevant data. We had four teams from Cambridge, Imperial College, Edinburgh, and Warrick. I gave the groups a couple of weeks to come up with models of disease spread. By that time,

MAFF became interested in what we were doing. Sir David King, the UK chief scientific advisor, became interested as well.

I held a meeting in late March in which the modelers presented their results. The government veterinary service came along. Neil Ferguson, from the Imperial Group, gave a lucid presentation in which he showed that the doubling time was nine days. Half of the animal farms in Britain would be affected by mid-May 2001. There was a stunned silence in the room. I asked Mark Woolhouse from Edinburgh about his results. He said that he had modeled the epidemic in a slightly different way, but his results were essentially the same. They agreed that a possible way to stop the spread was to develop a clean ring culling policy. The animals around an infected farm would have to be culled to create a buffer zone.

As the meeting broke up, David King decided to write to the prime minister immediately. There was one wrinkle; we had agreed that nothing would be said in public until MAFF was given an opportunity to digest the information. But that night Roy Anderson appeared on TV and spilled the beans. At that point, I stepped back, but David King continued to hold weekly meetings with the group. I went to a few of those meetings, but my role had been primarily to initiate the process.

There was a question that arose about the use of vaccines in the northern part of the country. Cattle are kept inside during the winter and then put out to pasture in early April to graze. The concern was that they would catch the disease and then have to be slaughtered. The thinking was that if they were vaccinated before, then they wouldn't have to be slaughtered, but the dairy and farming industries objected very strongly. They felt that the public would be concerned about the safety of the milk, and they had export concerns.

In early April, we met with Tony Blair at Chequers, his country residence, with the chief executives of supermarkets and with the president of the farmers' union. David King and Nick Brown attended as well. The industry was concerned about a crisis of consumer confidence if vaccines were used. The prime minister gave an eloquent speech and the industry consented, but the next day, they changed their minds. As a result, many more tens of thousands of cattle were destroyed.

Another concern that emerged was the fear that the massive funeral pyres of the burning animals would release dioxins, which are thought to be carcinogens, into the environment. If cattle ate dioxin-covered grass, there was, in theory, a risk that it could get into the milk supply.

We had a team looking at this through modeling. There were huge uncertainties. My answer was that we didn't think there was a problem, but we couldn't be sure. Supermarket milk is derived from milk mixed from many different areas; so if there were a problem, it would likely be diluted out. But with milk sold from local farms, we had to acknowledge our uncertainty.

The MAFF officials went ballistic when I said that. They said that I couldn't say this in public. They even told me that the prime minister would be unhappy with such an announcement. I went on TV anyway and made my announcement that we couldn't be certain about the safety of milk. Our advice was that supermarket milk would be okay, but local milk from [farms near] funeral pyres might not be. We also advised people what to do if they were worried.

Thank goodness, telling the truth had the exact opposite effect. There was no change in consumer confidence about milk. The media were happy that someone was finally telling them the truth. And in the end, when we tested the milk, there was no problem.

I believe that the modeling was immensely powerful in predicting the course of the epidemic. There was a lot of tension among the FMD virologists, the veterinarians, and the modelers. As far as I was concerned, the modelers never complained to me about their data. The veterinarians and virologists were unfamiliar with mathematical modeling. They are trained to treat patients, not to deal with population dynamics.

I think the overall response was good in the circumstances. We brought in the right experts to look at the problem. Through proper scientific analysis, we were able to change the government's perception of what needed to be done. The scientific results influenced the implementation of policy. I think it would have been much better too if the animals had been vaccinated, but the industry refused.

MAFF was in denial the crucial first four weeks of the epidemic. Had it implemented a movement restriction order on the sheep immediately, the epidemic would have taken a different course. MAFF learned that lesson during the 2007 outbreak when the FMD virus escaped from a laboratory. The outbreak was quickly contained.

Nick Brown, the minister of MAFF, lost his job as a result of the crisis. The prime minister and chief science advisor took the whole thing out of his hands. MAFF ceased to be a department and became DEFRA [Department for Environment, Food, and Rural Affairs]. I think it is important to not get seduced by your own convictions. It is important to get outside experts to give advice. Also, it is important to not forget lessons learned from previous crises. After 15 years, the ministers and civil servants are all new, and they don't know what happened in the past.[61]

Professor Alex Donaldson was head of Pirbright Laboratory of the Institute for Animal Health (IAH) from 1989 to 2002, during the FMD crisis. Here are his comments:

I was in charge of the Pirbright Laboratory during 2001 and so all of the activities concerning the laboratory were my responsibility. One of my first tasks was to respond to a request from Jim Scudamore, CVO, to visit the abattoir in Essex where suspected FMD had been reported. I examined the animals, confirmed that the clinical signs were typical of FMD, and told

Jim what I had seen. He officially reported an outbreak of FMD in the UK that evening.

During the next few days, colleagues from Pirbright who had expertise in FMD visited four farms located in the northeast, southwest, and east of the country to examine cases of FMD. They estimated the age of lesions, especially the oldest; performed epidemiological investigations; and collected samples for detailed laboratory investigations.

The laboratory determined by nucleotide sequencing that the causal virus belonged to the type O_1 pan-Asia group, and by antigenic analysis, that the most appropriate vaccine for emergency use would be one containing the O_1 Manisa strain. We also carried out experiments in animals to determine the virulence and transmissibility of the virus strain. We found that the risk of the strain being spread by the wind was low—much lower than that seen with the O_1 strain that caused the epidemic in the UK from 1967–68.

During the 2001 epidemic, Pirbright tested more than 15,400 diagnostic specimens for evidence of infection. Later the laboratory performed more than one million serological tests on blood samples looking for antibodies to the FMD virus to demonstrate that the UK was free from infection.

During and after the epidemic, we received more than 2,000 phone calls from the media and the public. At the start, I tried to handle most of them, but this soon became impossible and so many were dealt with by Professor Chris Bostock, director of IAH,[62] and also by Dr. Paul Kitching, who was my deputy.

When the first outbreak of FMD was reported on February 20, Nick Brown, minister of MAFF, was in charge. Early in the epidemic, the traditional, well-proven policies for eradicating the FMD virus were used successfully in Essex County. However, the disease spread more extensively in other parts of the country mainly because a severe personnel shortage constrained the control and eradication efforts.

In the middle of March, after Brown had made some public statements that the epidemic was under control, Tony Blair decided to sack him and take over. Blair remained in charge until the last outbreak on September 30.

Jim Scudamore's role initially was to advise Nick Brown on disease control policies and to direct their implementation by the State Veterinary Service. After Professor David King, chief scientific advisor, took over in the middle of March, he became responsible for disease control policy and Scudamore's role changed to merely directing the operational activities of the State Veterinary Service.

King was responsible for the 24/48-hour culling policy that was promoted by mathematical modelers and led by a Royal Society cartel.

The 24/48-hour cull policy was implemented on March 29, but this was after the epidemic had peaked and the number of outbreaks was already in decline. I had no problem with the 24-hour culling policy, which meant that infected animals were slaughtered within 24 hours of being identified. However, I did find fault with the 48-hour culling policy, which involved the culling within 48 hours of animals in farms neighboring infected premises (IPs)—on the assumption that they were infected.

However, this policy was not supported by clear scientific evidence. My view, and that of my veterinary colleagues at Pirbright, was that the only contiguous farms that should have been culled were those identified by epidemiological investigations as dangerous contact premises (DCs).[63] The stamping out of IPs and DCs is the traditional and well-proven way to eradicate FMD virus.

It is my view that the CVO should have remained in charge and not have been marginalized. An FMD specialist from Pirbright should have accompanied him when talking to the media to provide a more balanced and persuasive opinion. Traditional methods for controlling FMD work—you don't need unproven methodologies. The mathematical models used in 2001 were not validated, and studies performed since have shown that they complicated an already difficult situation.

The consequences of the 2001 epidemic were severe. Farmers suffered greatly—especially those in areas where movement restrictions lasted for months on end with no compensation. I have heard it stated that more than 50 farmers committed suicide during the crisis.

An enormous amount has been learned in the years since 2001. During the 2007 outbreak, I was reassured that the modelers were kept off the scene, and the outbreak was quickly contained. It reinforced my criticism of using models that have not been properly tested and validated.[64]

Dr. Joseph Anelli was a veterinarian with the U.S. Department of Agriculture (USDA) and director of emergency programs during the 2001 UK FMD eradication program. He assisted UK leaders during the crisis.

I was director of emergency programs at the USDA and, during the month of August 2001, I was based in MAFF headquarters on Page Street working with Dr. Scudamore and attending daily briefings. Early on, the size of the outbreak outstripped the UK's resources, and they were looking for veterinary help from other countries. My staff in the United States put together a group of 350 veterinarians and veterinary technicians to go to the UK on a rotational basis.

I closely watched what the UK was doing since there was a lot of concern that it might spread to the United States: we received around 450 calls per day. There was considerable confusion between hand-foot-mouth disease and FMD. People did not understand that hand-foot-mouth disease is a common viral respiratory infection of infants and children[65] and FMD is a deadly disease of livestock. People also confused the differences between FMD and BSE.

One Sunday, I got a phone call from a reporter who completely confused BSE and FMD. It takes months to get the results of a BSE test versus 24 to

48 hours for an FMD test. The reporter didn't understand this, and fortunately, I clarified the issue before the article was published.

The United States and the United Kingdom have systems in place for early identification of disease outbreaks. Veterinarians' licenses are contingent upon complying with rapid reporting of foreign animal diseases such as FMD and other deadly livestock diseases, since the effects of these diseases can be so great. We assume that when such a disease first shows up, it won't be hidden.

That wasn't the case in the UK. It took them awhile to figure out that a waste food feeder began feeding pigs raw waste because its cooker had broken down. People must be licensed and registered in order to properly cook waste for pigs. [Also] it's not clear if a ship from Africa or a local Asian restaurant illegally bringing in meat products led to the importation of the virus. Sick and dying hogs were sent to market and exposed sheep. By the time MAFF officials learned of the outbreak, the disease had spread all over the country. Its response plan had assumed that FMD would be detected very early and spread locally to as many as 10 farms. MAFF was well prepared for that scenario, but not for what actually happened.

The UK did not have enough people to respond quickly to get ahead of the disease. It took a month to get up to speed. As a result, Scudamore and others spent their time justifying what they were doing rather than simply getting the job done. It took resources away from controlling the disease, and, instead, put them into defending their approach. This struggle caused some policies to be put in place that might not have been best at controlling the disease.

The scientific reality was that the extent of the outbreak was unknown, but the political leadership didn't want maybes. There is a tendency to not assume a crisis is the worst case scenario or to report a negative or to give bad news. Government officials want to build confidence and to convey that things are under control.

Nick Brown was in charge, but his reassurances that things were under control—when they weren't—led to Blair's taking over. They had to decide which direction to go in the interface among scientific and technical information, public perceptions, and public messaging. We sometimes cause our own problems with public messaging when we get the initial messages wrong. If anything goes wrong, the perception is that it was not an honest mistake but incompetence. Officials are faulted if they thought of only the next step ahead instead of the next three steps. Political leadership tends to allow public opinion rather than science to drive policy.

People want immediate fixes for things. A maybe is not a definite yes or no. There are a lot of unknowns in disease outbreaks, and we're never right 100 percent of the time. The first time you're wrong, the media tears you apart, and then the next level of leadership steps in. I was once watching a news interview of a minister. I found out what our next policy would be because some reporter put him on the spot to make a statement about what he would do next.

The Royal Society's effort at mathematical modeling was an absolute disaster. Disease outbreaks almost follow chaos theory: there are many variables including human behavior that are impossible to predict. Prior to an outbreak, models can be very useful in developing preparedness policy, but there is no substitute for on the ground epidemiologic data to contain an outbreak.

Less than 5 percent of the total livestock in the UK were actually infected and/or slaughtered. The criticism came from those 5 percent of farmers whose livestock were already infected. MAFF had to protect the other 95 percent of the livestock, which included issuing permits for the movement of sheep. Since 95 percent of the sheep were healthy, they had to be allowed to graze on fresh pastures. Otherwise, they might as well have slaughtered 100 percent of the livestock. Allowing sheep to move to new pastures decreased the economic losses. This policy was in the best interest of the agriculture community even though it was the same activity that allowed the disease to spread in the first place.

When the political leadership turns over, the career civil servants have to reeducate a new group of leaders. It's easy to say that MAFF was the problem, so the political leaders did away with it and renamed it DEFRA. It will not necessarily be better. Many problems become cyclic. There is a reorganization of the original agency that was working in the first place, and then after 10 to 15 years, the same problems develop. It is difficult to interface political reality with a quick fix mentality.[66]

Sir Roy Anderson is professor of infectious diseases epidemiology in the Division of Epidemiology, Public Health and Primary Care at Imperial College, London. In 2000, he set up the program with a research team of around 40 people to study epidemiology, population biology, and evolution and control of infectious diseases such as HIV/AIDS, pandemic influenza, and BSE.

When the first few cases of foot-and-mouth disease trickled out, my research group started to work on the epidemiology of the outbreak. Normally, I work in the human area, but I have advised on veterinary issues such as BSE. I was skeptical when MAFF officials including the minister [Nick Brown] announced that the outbreak was "under control."

We have the world's leading groups in modeling infectious disease outbreaks. Outbreak modeling is largely based on one simple concept: the Basic Reproductive Number, "R_0." It is defined as the average number of secondary cases that develop from the primary case. For an epidemic to propagate, the value of R_0 must be greater than one. If R_0 is less than one, then the epidemic contracts.

We did an analysis based on the number of cases of FMD reported over time. It was quite obvious that R_0 was greater than one. We estimated that there would be an exponential rise in the number of cases and the epidemic was not as yet under control.

I was asked to come on *Newsnight,* BBC Television, to comment on Nick Brown's statement. When I said that the outbreak wasn't under control, a lot of questions were asked about the government stance. Then David King, the chief science advisor of the UK government, got involved and sought advice from the four best mathematical modeling groups in the UK to provide scientific analysis.

Our scientific analyses went smoothly and largely came to similar conclusions. We used Web-based data that the veterinarians entered in the field, so we had real-time data. The problem was that MAFF wasn't very good at analysis of the collected data. MAFF and the veterinary officials were very resistant to outsiders coming in. All four groups' analyses essentially showed the same thing: the animals had to be culled as fast as possible to get the epidemic under control.

Foot-and-mouth has a fast incubation time and spreads rapidly, infecting vast numbers of animals over wide areas. Speed is of the essence to get FMD under control; you have to cull animals as rapidly as possible post diagnosis. The culling policies were very controversial. MAFF was influenced by the farming and other communities that didn't want culling. There were transportation and tourism concerns. People were appalled at the slaughter of all the animals, and a lot of them came up with different solutions. All of the scientists, myself included, would have preferred a different, more humane solution. But speedy and draconian actions saved more animal lives in the long term than if the epidemic had not been brought under control.

The chief science advisor presented our data at the daily crisis meetings. After the first few weeks of the outbreak, Tony Blair took charge and chaired the meetings. It was an election year, so there were other things going on. Even without the distractions of high media interest, command and control can be difficult. But once Blair brought in the Ministry of Defense, things changed enormously. The military provided its logistics expertise.

Good leadership requires bringing in outside experts. Government departments fight like terriers to keep their domains. If a problem crosses department lines, as it did with FMD, collaboration across government departments can be difficult.

The FMD virologists were not the best people to give advice on the epidemiology and control of the epidemic. They prefer to put people in a room and get a consensus opinion. The veterinary and medical sciences have been slow to adapt to modern methods. We base our recommendations on computer analysis using calculations, analysis, and simulations. Our advice worked, and the epidemic was brought under control.[67]

France imported thousands of sheep from the UK before FMD was detected. The country faced a potential disaster, yet it managed to contain the crisis to two small outbreaks. Dr. Isabelle Chmitelin was the French CVO between 2000 and 2005. During this period, she faced the BSE crisis, the FMD crisis, and the avian influenza crisis in 2002.

My role as CVO involved three different levels: the European [EU] level, the national level, and the local level. At the EU level, I was involved in discussions and negotiations with the CVOs of the other member states and with the European Commission [EC] to set up adapted rules for animal movement inside the European community. At the national and local levels, I was involved in defining measures to be implemented on French territory and in implementing and coordinating the actions of local veterinary services.

At the national level, I was the first one informed about the situation in the UK. Early one morning, I got a direct call from Jim Scudamore's assistant, Robin Bell, who told me, "We identified outbreaks of FMD in the UK. You should also be infected."

Our first reaction was to assess the risk of exposure and to define the measures to be applied to control the risk. We realized through our computerized animal identification system that we had received about 20,000 sheep from the UK during the risk period. In addition, there was a Muslim religious festival [Eid al-Adha] going on that required families to slaughter their own sheep, so sheep were all over the country. FMD had potentially spread all over France. Quick decisions were necessary.

In France, veterinary services are under the supervision of the minister of agriculture who takes into account the political aspects. As CVO, I had to discuss the situation with the different ministerial departments and advise about the best technical measures to take. It was difficult because I had to discuss highly technical matters with people who didn't know a word about biology in general and FMD in particular.

You must be aware that FMD occurred just after BSE. So the ministers would ask me if FMD infected humans. When I said, "No," then they didn't care. I had to convince them that this was important. As a technical person, I was aware of the implications of the disease. The challenge was to convince the politicians that decisions needed to be made quickly!

I told the agriculture minister that we had to kill 50,000 sheep within the week. We had no legal basis to order such a massive slaughter, so we had to be sure that all the professional organizations agreed with the policy. We got approval from the farm organizations. Some of them were aware of the dangerous situation.

In the hierarchy of command, there was the minister of agriculture, the director of food safety, and me. The director of food safety was a woman whom I used to work with. She wasn't a veterinarian, but she was really well connected with the minister. That was the key to our success. She had confidence in me, and she served as a screen between the minister and me. Everything went quickly and smoothly.

In France, we have a very centralized chain of command. There is one chain of command from the local director of veterinary services to the national level. It is not like the federal system in the United States; it is very efficient. Also, it was much easier for us to deal with the disease because we had time. We had a computerized animal identification/movement database that was implemented in 1993 after the abolition of borders. I wasn't sure if all the animals were tagged and that we would find them. In the end, we were lucky.

The UK's detections system failed, so it identified the disease very late. It had to run after the disease. I'm not sure we would have done much better under those circumstances. When we killed 50,000 animals, we sampled their blood and found that six animals were positive. They were in all parts of France. If we had not killed them, we would not have been successful at containing FMD to two outbreaks.

France had two outbreaks: one in Normandy and the other in the Paris suburbs. The second was in direct connection to the first. The Muslim festival brought sheep into the Paris suburbs. Because of the festival, there were people arranging for sheep purchases and deliveries who normally do not handle such matters. This complicated the animal-tracking process.

Our biggest challenge involved the media and politics. It is difficult dealing with the media and managing crises in short time frames. You must be transparent, but the media want spectacular images. Also, the farmers wanted to see what was going on, so they would go to the problem sites and then go back to their farms. In the process, they potentially contaminated their farms.

If we had not reacted quickly to the outbreaks, we would have had a big problem with the public reaction. The public wanted vaccination, which makes a worse situation. There is no difference between vaccinated and infected animals.

Finally, you need to be supported by good professionals and good scientists. There must be confidence in the people above and below the chain of command. If decision making needs to be discussed, then it is not efficient. At the end of the day, it will be too late.[68]

SUMMING UP

Leaders during the 2001 FMD outbreak in the UK faced a difficult situation because the disease was not detected until after it had already spread around the country. The situation was exacerbated by shortages of personnel and resources: MAFF was not equipped for a disaster of this magnitude. In the early stages of the crisis, the agency's response was slow and ineffective in culling animals within 24 hours of diagnosis.

As with the early stages of the BSE crisis, MAFF officials initially downplayed the severity and spread of the FMD crisis. Nick Brown, the minister of MAFF, falsely reassured the public that the crisis was under control when, in fact, it was not. His reassurances undermined his credibility. Jim Scudamore, the CVO, was removed from primary control of the epidemic because he failed to have MAFF properly implement the 24-hour cull policy. By not killing and disposing of the animal carcasses within 24 hours, the outbreak became much harder to contain. These failures set into motion the change in leadership that itself made an already difficult situation worse.

Besides the communication failures giving false reassurances to the farmers and public that everything was under control, there were additional communication failures between government and industry. MAFF did not obtain the agriculture industry's full support of its response policies. On the contrary, farmers were rioting in opposition to the slaughter policies. The National Farmers' Union accused government officials of unfairly blaming farmers for the crisis.

There were communication failures between government agencies. For example, MAFF and Department of the Environment officials argued over animal movements, burial sites, and EU regulations. Rather than welcoming the logistical help from the Department of Defense, Nick Brown, the MAFF minister, complained that the military was taking over.

There were communication failures and competition between scientific experts, including the battle between FMD virologists and the mathematical modelers. As recognized FMD experts, both Dr. Kitching and Dr. Donaldson expressed anger and frustration by having their advice and authority usurped by Sir Roy Anderson and other mathematical modelers. The mathematical modelers believed that the slaughter policies their models supported were crucial to getting the epidemic under control. The pros and cons of using mathematical models during outbreaks are beyond the scope of this book; however, it is important to note that precious time was spent figuring out how to respond to the growing epidemic.

Tony Blair responded to political pressures by replacing Nick Brown and putting himself in charge of the FMD crisis. David King, the chief science advisor, replaced Jim Scudamore. Blair centralized decision making and dispatched the military to help with logistics and personnel shortages. He implemented the controversial 24/48-hour cull policy that included killing healthy animals on contiguous farms. This new extreme cull policy pushed farmers into revolt against the government's actions.

In the weeks leading up to the election, Blair worked hard to remove the FMD crisis from the public's eye. He relaxed the contiguous cull policy at the end of April and opened as much of the countryside to tourism as possible. Writing in *Parliamentary Affairs,* Allan McConnell and Alastair Stark asserted that Blair's relaxing of FMD containment policies because of politics prolonged the crisis until the end of September. Despite the considerable loss of animal life and the economic and social costs, however, the Blair government successfully managed to be reelected for a second term.[69]

MAFF's reputation was tarnished by the BSE crisis, but its abysmal handling of the FMD crisis led to its dissolution and replacement by a new agency, the Department for Environment, Food, and Rural Affairs (DEFRA). This new agency's approach would be one of transparency and cooperation rather than the secrecy, departmentalism, and defensive decision making that characterized MAFF. Centralization would replace fragmentation.[70]

In contrast to the disorganized and slow UK response, France's decision making was centralized with a simple chain of command involving three people: the agriculture minister, the director of food safety, and the CVO. The director of food safety and the CVO had a good working relationship built on trust that facilitated communication with the agriculture minister. Even so, Chmitelin recounted how she had to convince the agriculture minister that FMD was important even though humans could not be infected. France had additional advantages in that the crisis was recognized early, and the country had a computerized animal-tracking system facilitating the identification of animals that had been imported from the UK. The response was rapid, effective, and limited to 50,000 animals.

CONCLUSION

Political and bureaucratic leaders responding to animal health crises need to recognize that directly or indirectly, humans will be affected. In the case of BSE, the prion could infect both animals and people. The fear of possibly being infected caused considerable human distress. Although FMD infected only animals, people were severely affected economically, socially, and psychologically.

Since 1940, the number of infectious diseases emerging from animals to infect humans has increased.[71] These diseases have included BSE, HIV/AIDS, Hendra and Nipah viruses, Severe Acute Respiratory Syndrome (SARS), and West Nile virus. As humans continue to disturb fragile ecosystems and implement intensive agricultural practices, leaders should anticipate that more diseases will emerge. During the initial stages of such crises, there will be little, if any, scientific knowledge to support policy decisions.

Decision making will require scientific advice from many disciplines, including veterinary medicine, human medicine, public health, epidemiology, molecular biology, ecology, business, communications, and international relations. As the BSE and FMD crises demonstrated, leaders must choose their scientific advisors carefully. Independent scientists with potential conflicts of interest might be faulted for giving biased or self-serving advice. On the other hand, government scientists, even if they are recognized experts, might be viewed with suspicion simply because of their insider status—as occurred with FMD experts Kitching and Donaldson.

Scientific advisory committees hastily set up to handle a crisis might not function as effectively as longstanding committees in which scientists spend time learning to communicate with one another. As described by Dr. Manuguerra in chapter 6, longstanding committees benefit from the perspectives of scientists from a variety of disciplines. Scientists should feel free to disagree with one another as they deliberate and not be exposed to public scrutiny until after they draw reasonably firm conclusions with background supportive data made available for unbiased criticism.

Complicated crises involving animals such as livestock require careful and effective communications among government agencies, industry, the media, and the public. Experts such as veterinarians and research scientists must be able to communicate with one another, with elected officials, with industry representatives, and with the public. Their education and training might not necessarily include communication skills. There should be more leadership training in medical, veterinary medical, and schools of public health to prepare these professionals to work effectively under crisis conditions.

If an animal health crisis is caused by a zoonotic agent, such as avian influenza, BSE, or West Nile virus, then leaders from both human and animal health need to work together to contain the spread of the disease. During much of the 20th century, collaborative efforts between human and animal health experts were limited. The infrastructure of government agencies illustrates this point. Departments of agriculture focus on livestock health even though the health of livestock can affect humans. Departments of health focus solely on human health even though human health is influenced by environmental factors. These agencies do not typically work with each other.

The animal health crises described in this chapter illustrate the challenges leaders face when trying to bridge animal and human health. MAFF's mission was to promote agriculture and oversee animal health. Its mission did not include human health even though the BSE and FMD crises very much impacted human health and well-being. As Dr. Meldrum indicated, no one, neither MAFF nor health department officials, wanted to discuss food safety with the media.

Communication and collaboration with the human health sector were not seamless. As the BSE crisis persisted, MAFF eventually reached out to the Department of Health, which recommended that an advisory group be formed to address the risk of BSE to humans. Surveillance for CJD revealed that humans were getting sick and dying from eating affected meat products.

During the FMD crisis, humans were affected economically, socially, and psychologically. Farmers and their families might have benefited from prompt social services to prevent feelings of isolation and suicidal ideation. Instead, a number of farmers committed suicide.

There is a growing "One Health" movement that recognizes the interconnectedness among human, animal, and environmental health and seeks to increase integration, communication, collaboration, and cooperation among the various disciplines, including human and veterinary medicine.[72] Implementing "One Health" would require government agencies to work differently. They would have to build better bridges to work with one another, or they would have to be reorganized to facilitate improved crossspecies and environmental disease surveillance, prevention, and control programs.

Regardless of how government agencies are organized to address these challenges, what is important is that joint efforts between leaders in human and animal health would be critical in the rapid identification and response to outbreaks involving both human and animal populations. Leaders in animal health must have the same level of authority and decision making as their human counterparts. Veterinarians and physicians must work as colleagues and be integral parts of the chains of command. These chains of command could be integrated or work in parallel, but they would have to address both animal and human health crises to achieve better health for all.

Chapter 8

REACHING THE MASSES

Threats to public health are communicated with astonishing speed in today's information age. When threats are real and immediate, leaders need to plan communication strategies carefully and use the appropriate media to convey them. Successful messages are often simple and repetitive.

Problems arise when leaders ignore or hide a crisis, downplay the severity of a crisis, provide false reassurances, or give misleading or inaccurate information. Journalists prefer to get information from scientists and medical professionals who can provide up-to-date information on the crisis at hand. These professionals, however, tend to use technical jargon and are not necessarily good communicators. Elected officials might be good communicators but tend to give false reassurances or misinformation. Together, these traits contribute to leadership confusion by frustrating journalists and unnecessarily misleading the public. Regardless of who does the communicating, journalists play a critical role in disseminating information.

RISK ASSESSMENT, PERCEPTION, AND COMMUNICATION

When their lives are threatened, people experience fear, anger, anxiety, and denial. Such strong emotions can change how people perceive their environment and impair their decision-making ability. Compromised decision-making capabilities can lead to ineffective or, worse, counterproductive actions.[1] The leader's challenge during a crisis is to inform the public effectively of known risks, and how to avoid them, without inciting panic.

The challenge in advising people of possible harm comes from the inherent uncertainty of the risks. No one can predict the future, so the chance that a threat will actually manifest has to be communicated as a probability (the relative likelihood that something will occur). For most people, probability is a difficult concept to grasp.

Effective communication is further complicated because it requires that leaders understand how people think about and respond to risk. The field of *risk assessment* aims to improve how we identify, characterize, and quantify risk.[2] It does so by incorporating the psychological study of how humans perceive risk (i.e., *risk perception*).

Studies have shown that risk means different things to different people; technical experts judge risk differently than does the lay public, for example. Technical experts typically include annual fatality rates in their estimates of risk, whereas the lay public places greater emphasis on subjective factors such as perceived lack of control, catastrophic potential, and fatal consequences.[3] Some experts believe the lay public perceives potential hazards as either *safe* or *risky*.[4] Safe hazards are those that are familiar and voluntary and can be controlled by the individual, such as driving a car, smoking a cigarette, drinking alcohol, or owning a handgun.[5] In contrast, the use of nuclear power and flying in an airplane are seen as risky because they are unfamiliar, controlled by others, and generally not voluntary—even though fewer people die from nuclear accidents and airplane crashes per year than from the perceived safe hazards.[6]

The field of risk communication developed in the mid-1980s.[7] Risk communication is a scientific approach to communicating effectively in crisis situations; it combines elements of conflict resolution, health education, psychology, public affairs, and both risk assessment and risk perception.[8] Applied carefully, its goal is to help people keep their fears in perspective and allow them to continue making reasonable, rational decisions even under stress.[9] Communicating risk is challenging in other ways when a crisis is in progress, however, because the hazards are real and immediate.

In the fall of 2001, elected officials and public health professionals struggled to communicate with one another and with the public during the anthrax attacks. Tommy Thompson, U.S. Secretary of Health and Human Services, suggested to the media that the case of inhalational anthrax in Florida might have occurred naturally. Dr. Larry Bush, the physician treating the initial victim, was shocked by Thompson's statement because Bush believed the patient was almost certainly a victim of a deliberate bioterrorist attack.[10]

The U.S. Centers for Disease Control and Prevention (CDC), the federal agency responsible for investigating the crisis, remained largely silent as the media clamored for information.[11] Dr. Jeffrey Koplan, CDC director, and his staff were accused of being inaccessible and of not providing enough information to the public.[12] Koplan later wrote about his experience:

> Taking time out to face the microphones diverts public health practitioners from their functions and responsibilities during a major crisis. . . . That calculus may have shifted forever with the anthrax attacks of 2001. . . . It became obvious that public communication had become in some sense fully as important as—if not even more important than—the line duties of senior decision makers.[13]

Thompson was criticized for political grandstanding by providing technical information that was expected to come from a physician. Koplan announced his resignation in February 2002, six months after the anthrax letters were first mailed.[14]

In response to the difficulties that government officials encountered during the anthrax attacks, Barbara Reynolds, CDC Office of Communication, and Matthew Seeger, Department of Communication at Wayne State University, developed a model that integrated risk communication with crisis response called, "Crisis and Emergency Risk Communication (CERC)."[15] In contrast to risk communication, which focuses on conveying potential risk factor probabilities, CERC addresses what is known or not known about a specific event as well as the potential risks to the public. CERC seeks to reduce the inherent uncertainties of crises by assuming that most crises will evolve in predictable ways: risk, eruption, cleanup and recovery, and evaluation.[16] Of course, the authors recognize that many disasters are not always so predictable, especially if the crisis involves something novel, such as a previously unknown infectious agent.

Who delivers the message is as important as the message itself. For example, the public is more likely to believe a message if it is given by someone with credibility. If the messenger has a reputation for previous misrepresentation, self-serving framing of messages, or professional incompetence, the public may discount the message being given, even if it is otherwise believable.[17] Once an individual has lost his or her credibility, it is very hard to regain it. For example, during the FMD crisis described in chapter 7, Part II, Nick Brown, the MAFF minister, and Jim Scudamore, the CVO, lost their credibility after giving false reassurances, and subsequently lost their positions of authority.

Presciently, crisis communication strategies were used to great effect during the 1947 smallpox outbreak in New York City.

SMALLPOX OUTBREAK IN NEW YORK CITY, 1947

In February 1947, a 47-year-old merchant named Eugene Le Bar and his wife boarded a bus in Mexico bound for New York City.[18] The bus made stops in Texas, Missouri, Ohio, and Pennsylvania, and arrived in New York City on March 1.[19] By that time, Le Bar was not feeling well, but despite his illness, he and his wife explored New York City by sightseeing and shopping in several large department stores.[20] With a fever of 105 degrees and an odd rash on his face and hands, he entered the dermatology ward at Bellevue Hospital on March 5. Smallpox was not diagnosed because he had previously had a smallpox vaccination, and he denied exposure to the disease.[21]

When his condition deteriorated, Le Bar was transferred to the Willard Parker Hospital, the city's communicable disease hospital, on March 8. Doctors believed he was suffering from an adverse drug reaction because he had been taking several painkillers, including one that causes rashes in certain people.[22] After two days of delirium, he died on March 10.[23]

Three individuals who were hospitalized at Willard Parker Hospital at the same time as Le Bar subsequently developed smallpox. Physicians reexamined Le Bar's chart and concluded that he must have been the initial smallpox case. Dr. Dorothea Tolle, medical superintendent of Willard Parker Hospital, called the New York City Health Department to notify it that there was a possible smallpox outbreak.[24] Pus taken from the patients' rashes was sent for analysis to the Army Medical Center laboratory in Washington, D.C., one of only two laboratories in the country equipped to diagnose smallpox;[25] the reports came back positive for smallpox on April 4.

Mayor William O'Dwyer had appointed Dr. Israel Weinstein as New York City's commissioner of health the previous year.[26] The same day that he learned of the smallpox diagnosis, Weinstein announced the outbreak to the public.[27] He estimated that between 5,000 and 10,000 individuals were at risk of becoming infected with smallpox, given Le Bar's itinerary.[28]

Weinstein notified the U.S. Public Health Service of the outbreak. He then spoke with Dr. Edward Bernecker, New York City commissioner of hospitals, and convened the administrative officers of the Departments of Health and Hospitals to formulate a response plan and strategy.[29] He presented the facts to Mayor O'Dwyer, who agreed that an intensive vaccination campaign was needed to control the outbreak; Weinstein would organize, direct, and administer the citywide containment effort.[30] The mayor would provide political support.

Karl Pretshold, chief of public relations, and Caroline Sulzer, assistant in health education of the New York City Department of Health, realized that there was no time to plan a step-by-step publicity campaign or to develop and administer a public health education program to address the crisis. But they had two important advantages: the Health Department had a sterling reputation among New Yorkers, and the public relations team in the Health Department had ready access to key decision makers. In addition, they cultivated the confidence and cooperation of city newspapers and radio stations.[31]

Weinstein began a two-part containment effort: a mass vaccination program and an intensive campaign to identify all those who were potentially exposed to the disease. He announced that anyone in the city who had not been vaccinated since early childhood should get vaccinated immediately.[32] When speaking to the press, Weinstein chose his words carefully so as not to incite public panic. His message was simple and clear, "Be safe. Be sure. Get vaccinated."[33]

The outbreak made front page news after a second death from smallpox occurred. Mayor O'Dwyer urged his fellow citizens to get vaccinated while he received the vaccine from Weinstein. The mayor said:

> I have consulted with Dr. Weinstein and Dr. Thomas Rivers of the Board of Health, a leading world authority in this field. They think that all the city's available medical machinery and manpower should be thrown into this situation to vaccinate everyone in the city within the next three weeks.[34]

The Health Department press office made sure that the people covering the story understood that they had a responsibility to help with the vaccination campaign and to avoid panicking the public. Every reporter who interviewed Weinstein was vaccinated. Special squads of physicians were sent to vaccinate newspaper editors and staff while they were on the job.[35]

The Health Department had a positive relationship with the media because of its policy of responding to reporters' queries quickly and candidly. This policy kept frightening stories, gossip, and rumors to a minimum since reporters would routinely check with the Health Department to verify reports or leads from other sources. As a result, only one rumor was reported as fact when a story had been printed before the reporter had confirmed it with the Health Department.[36]

The Health Department placed its Bureau of Laboratories on an emergency work schedule to package 250,000 doses of smallpox vaccine.[37] Despite this, supplies of the vaccine ran out. Rather than focusing on the shortage—which could have derailed the vaccination campaign—newspapers instead reported on how the mayor had solved the shortage by quickly securing thousands of additional units from the U.S. Army and

Navy.[38] The mayor addressed the city's long-term needs by putting pressure on drug companies to make more vaccine available and sell it to the city more cheaply.[39]

The press played a key role in fostering the public's sense of civic duty and willingness to volunteer. In addition to its regular workforce, the Health Department depended on thousands of volunteers to help at almost 180 special clinics set up to provide the vaccine free of charge. This campaign was aided by the many wartime volunteers who were still available, including those from the American Red Cross and the American Women's Voluntary Services.[40]

In less than a month, more than 6 million people were vaccinated. Only 12 people came down with smallpox, and 2 died.[41] Despite problems in the campaign, including approximately 46 cases of encephalitis and 8 deaths resulting from adverse vaccine effects, the response was hailed as a success.[42] The members of the Health Department's public relations department were instrumental in the effort; they emphasized giving the press the facts and then explaining what they were doing and why they were doing it.[43]

The 1947 New York City smallpox outbreak response has been considered a model effort.[44] Despite the adverse reactions to the vaccine (more people died from adverse vaccine reactions than from smallpox), the outbreak was contained with great media and public support. Without credible, effective leadership and widespread support from the press and the public, civil unrest and considerable human suffering and death could have resulted.

In contrast, a smallpox outbreak in Milwaukee, Wisconsin, 53 years earlier resulted in street riots. In that outbreak, the press gave mixed, partisan messages and limited information. Poor people were forced into isolation hospitals, whereas the wealthy were allowed to stay in their homes under voluntary quarantine and isolation. In addition, the public did not understand the importance of vaccination, and the health department did not do a public education campaign.[45] The end result was disaster: more than 1,000 Milwaukeeans came down with smallpox and 244 died.

These two examples, New York and Milwaukee, illustrate the differences in public perception and response when effective crisis risk communication is used and when it is not. In New York, effective crisis risk communication was used to great effect. People understood the crisis and volunteered to help and to get vaccinated. In Milwaukee, crisis risk communication was not used, but rather, ineffective and partisan messages were given. The result was public rioting and unnecessary deaths.

Not only were New York City officials effective in crisis risk communication, but it is also important to note that the leadership roles of the mayor and health commissioner were clearly delineated and complementary. In this scenario, Mayor O'Dwyer provided political support for

Dr. Weinstein's decisions, essentially following the Glendening Model of crisis leadership described in chapter 5. These two individuals worked well together using this model.

Weinstein had the credibility to make the decision to mass vaccinate the entire New York City population. He and his public relations team intuitively used effective, simple, and repetitive language with the press to educate the public about the importance of vaccination, and they quickly responded to all queries with factual, nonpolitical messages. Unknowingly, they implemented CERC almost sixty years before the concept was formalized.[46]

THE CHANGING MEDIA

Of course, in 1947, the United States was an optimistic nation. Working together with its international allies, it had just won World War II. The press and the public trusted the government. It was an era before the Vietnam War, Watergate, the Iraq War, and Hurricane Katrina, events that led to increasing distrust of public officials.

Can an outbreak communication effort be conducted successfully in a world with widespread public cynicism toward government? How might the media of the 21st century affect public sentiment and cooperation during an epidemic? Media outlets are no longer limited to newspapers, magazines, and radio but now include network, cable and satellite television, and the Internet. Information is available 24 hours a day, 7 days a week.

The U.S. media have also changed their approach to journalism: the line between news and entertainment has become blurred.[47] In 1968, CBS launched the TV newsmagazine *60 Minutes,* which conducted responsible investigative reporting. Tabloid television news programs, which started in the 1980s with *Entertainment Tonight,* began to change the nature of news by presenting celebrity gossip in a news format. *A Current Affair, Hard Copy,* and *Inside Edition* followed and were essentially TV versions of supermarket tabloids conducting sensationalistic journalism. Television newscasts began adopting some of the characteristics of these tabloid news shows in an effort to boost their ratings. Over time, the media have become increasingly less objective reporters of news and more active shapers of the news to make it as appealing as possible.[48]

Some go so far as to claim that the media have become entirely superficial, biased, and sensationalistic. These shortcomings are exacerbated by politicians' well-known use of spin when communicating, further diminishing public trust. Such practices, and the failure to involve the public when planning and executing a crisis response, increase the risk of social disruption during an epidemic. Experts propose that journalism should have clear reporting standards that must be followed during such crises: knowledge and facts are counters to sensationalism and super-ficiality.[49]

The media is no longer the sole source of crisis communications. The public can now share their personal experiences and opinions with each other on a global scale. Unfortunately, during the 2009 swine flu pandemic, social networking sites such as Twitter helped fuel public fears. People sent out endless barrages of short messages called "tweets" in hyperbolic language in order to get attention during the crisis. Since anyone, not just journalists, can communicate on these social networking sites, unsubstantiated facts, rumors, and personal opinions can spread and misinform others.[50] This new twist in crisis communications has forced public officials to be creative. For example, the CDC began a Twitter following called CDCemergency.[51]

FROM THE MEDIA PERSPECTIVE

The modern journalist must balance a number of contesting factors when reporting, such as competition between media outlets, the shifting interests of news consumers, and the private interests of those providing information to be reported.

To examine outbreak responses from the media's perspective, the three crises described in chapters 4 and 5 (anthrax, cryptosporidium, and Severe Acute Respiratory Syndrome–SARS) are examined here. Three newspaper reporters, a television news reporter, and a director of news and public affairs of a local public television station were interviewed regarding their experiences and opinions during the crises. The interviews appear in the following sections.

ANTHRAX OUTBREAK IN NEW JERSEY, 2001

Mark Perkiss is a former reporter with the *Trenton Times:*

> My involvement in the crisis began when the story initially broke. My goal was to provide as much information as possible. I had to go to as many people as I could, including politicians, to find out what the situation was. Initially people didn't know what was going on. There was something about a tainted letter. I asked, "Who's at risk? Is there a risk to anyone else?" Different officials had different opinions with conflicting views. There was a lot of not knowing and not understanding by the police, public health, etc.
>
> I don't think there is a difference in roles between print, television, and radio during a crisis. There is a difference in the approach, but the goals are the same. Newspapers are able to explain things more fully. Television

and radio condense information to a sound bite—whatever time is allotted. Newspapers have much more space.

I think there is a natural reaction to not want to give bad news, but it is important to state what the reality is. I understand that there is a line that people don't want to cross to [inadvertently] panic people. Officials and reporters don't want to panic people, but trying not to cross a line builds in friction. Overall, I think the more forthcoming, the better it is.[52]

Bill Jobes was director of news and public affairs for the public television station New Jersey Network News:

I was the chief journalist for the network. I decided who's assigned and what's covered. I edited the script. We have an advantage over commercial television in that public television does more in-depth coverage of the news. We covered the public health, police, and postal service briefings. The anthrax story went on for months, and we followed the story, including the remediation of the [contaminated] Hamilton postal facility.

The roles between print and television media are markedly different, and with the onset of multiple media news, the role of television has changed. The public is accustomed to a multitude of news sources. I don't think television is as important as it was 20 years ago. The public can become quickly aware of critical information, which is a good thing, but the media can go overboard. Stories continue to get coverage until the next obsession occurs. It is good for society as a whole, but when Homeland Security ratchets up terror alerts to keep us on edge—that's the downside.

Glen Gilmore [the mayor of Hamilton Township] became a celebrity during the anthrax crisis, which is okay at a certain level. We in the media prefer to talk to the professionals, the physicians and scientists, who can really tell us what is going on. We would call public relations at the state health department several times per day and would be referred down the chain usually to the professionals who know something. The problem is many of these professionals are muzzled by the elected officials. Whenever there is news, they [elected officials] want to manage it, spin it, and control it. Our job is to plow through it all and figure out what is going on. The full story is rarely told. Reporters are usually aware of being "spun," particularly those of us who report hard news. We are familiar with it.

We prefer to deal with people with credibility, such as someone with a long track record, and we expect a reasonable amount of information. Some reporters, particularly those who used to work in government agencies, are closer than others to the power brokers. But reporters are always skeptical, and they are more skeptical now than they were 25 years ago, particularly in Washington, D.C. I was in Washington during the Watergate hearings; the skepticism is far deeper now.

In general, reporters need to do their homework and understand the story. I read a lot of newspapers every day. They give you the ability to digest information that television doesn't. Anthrax was a very complicated story with many components, and especially [hard to cover fully] on a television deadline. There were a multitude of agencies across local, state, and federal jurisdictions. It was hard to get everything right.[53]

CRYPTOSPORIDIUM OUTBREAK
IN WISCONSIN, 1993

Donald Behm was a reporter with the *Milwaukee Journal:*

I was one of the three primary reporters during the outbreak for the *Milwaukee Journal.* At the time, there were two separate papers, the *Journal* and the *Sentinel.* The merger of the papers came several years later.

I divide the outbreak into two periods of time: before the boil water order and after the boil water order. Before the boil water order, the cause of the outbreak was unknown. There were a lot of anecdotes of widespread illnesses. There were photos of stores and pharmacies running out of [anti-diarrheal] medications. It was frustrating for the public and media because there were no explanations of the cause from health officials and hospitals. We asked the Milwaukee Water Works officials if it was the water, and they just refused to even consider water as a source of the illness. Officials never disclosed the inability to effectively remove particles—not to Nannis [the city health commissioner], the mayor, or the media. Prior to the boil water order, there was panic developing in the city. There were school closures. Businesses had huge numbers of people out sick.

At the press conference when the mayor announced the boil water order, he and Nannis were careful to not point fingers at the Water Works. I thought it was appropriate that the mayor issue the boil water order. The order was described as a precaution, but one of the local doctors had confirmed cryptosporidiosis in several of his patients. Officials were still drawing back from placing blame. By the next day, there were stories about stores running out of bottled water and restaurants boiling huge pots of water for use. The images of a large American city boiling its drinking water were frequently described as being similar to [those from] a third-world [country]. Once the mayor announced the boil water order, the media's role was investigational. What went wrong? What happened? No one in Milwaukee was familiar with cryptosporidium. We had to explain the symptoms of the infection and lack of medical treatment, etc.

Television gave this outbreak a lot of time, but it focused on dramatic images of the first few days. The print side took it a step further. In two days, I had a story about what went wrong at the South Side (Howard Ave.) water treatment plant. I was familiar with treatment plant operations. I had been reporting on studies of lead in drinking water here.

Prior to the outbreak, there was a lot of complacency in the Milwaukee Water Works—little was done to maintain or upgrade the water treatment plants. There was a lot of divisive interdepartmental politics. The Water Works didn't share its water problems with the public health officials. Nannis expressed frustration.

What reporters should have done before the boil water order was issued was bypass the wall of denial and go to outside water quality and disease outbreak experts. Immediately after the boil water order, I called several researchers around the country. Several of those researchers subsequently were also used by the city to help focus public and Milwaukee Common Council [a legislative body consisting of 15 members who represent the 15 districts of the city] attention on how to treat water that might contain cryptosporidium.

Now all media routinely turn to outside experts for comment on a local crisis or problem. Milwaukee media had been complacent too long, and dependent on local sources. We had never been confronted with an outbreak of this size and also had not been confronted with local officials who couldn't or wouldn't explain what was going on.[54]

SARS OUTBREAK IN TORONTO, 2003

Andre Picard was a public health reporter for the *Globe and Mail* during the 2003 SARS outbreak:

The *Globe and Mail* is a big national newspaper based in Toronto. My role, as a public health reporter, is to step back, give context and perspective, rather than body counts. The SARS crisis was like a feeding frenzy. It was treated like a plane crash.

There was a public health crisis team of four physicians doing daily, sometimes twice daily, press conferences. The four physicians were Colin D'Cunha [Ontario commissioner of public health], James Young [Ontario commissioner of public safety], Donald Low [chief microbiologist of Mount Sinai Hospital, Toronto], and Sheela Basrur [Toronto medical officer of health]. We called them the four physicians of the apocalypse. They would say things like, "Today two more people died." They weren't providing context. The numbers were presented in a cumulative fashion. They could have taken it one step further and presented an epidemic curve. The question, "Where are we at?" didn't get answered until later as a retrospective.

The daily briefings of these four were all very tightly controlled. There was no access to the hospitals since they were shut down, so trying to get a story by talking to people in hospital was not an option.

Colin D'Cunha was a toady for government. The others didn't agree with him. There was a lot of backroom political fighting. As a reporter, it wasn't clear to me who was in charge. Nobody was enough in charge. There needed to be clearer leadership since there was confusion with the four of them talking. I thought Dr. Basrur was the best of the four at providing good information. Donald Low became the media face.

There should have been one principal messenger. The message wasn't given well.

The public health officials became tourism promoters. This was appropriate for the politicians, but not for public health. The lines [of responsibility] have to be clear.

It was appropriate for politicians to focus on the economic impact of the outbreak since the WHO travel advisory was harming Toronto. This added to the hysteria.

Richard Schabas, the Ontario medical officer of health before D'Cunha, was chief of staff of York Central Hospital, which was the first SARS hospital. He was a voice in the wilderness and got crapped upon a lot.

I thought the Ontario health minister, Tony Clement, did a good job.[55] He was in a no-win position. He was at a baseball game when he got a call about the outbreak. He got a lot of flak for being at the game. He went and visited a hospital. I thought he did well and gave a balanced message. He didn't have a health background, but he knew his stuff.

[Toronto Mayor] Lastman was better not around. He was on *Larry King Live* and denounced WHO. He was a buffoon. He played a small role since health is a provincial [responsibility].

Culture and language played a big role in this outbreak. There was another parallel story in the Toronto Chinese-language papers. Since we had a Chinese translator, we were able to read the stories. The Chinese community felt singled out, and there was confusion between health and economics.

Newspapers need to invest in people who can understand these complex stories. It is a failing of the media for not having trained reporters who can provide context. Crime scene reporters often get thrown into covering these stories. The media coverage reached a frenzy when the outbreak curve was on the way down.[56]

Maureen Taylor was a national health/medical reporter for CBC Television News during the SARS outbreak:

I didn't see my role [as being] any different from any other news reporter. The [disease] was brand new. We didn't know what we were dealing with. We were reporting in the absence of knowledge and were trying not to be alarmist. It was trying to get my bosses interested in the story because it was occurring at the same time as the U.S. invasion of Iraq. At first, I had to fight to get the story on the news.

The public health officials wanted the media to get their messages out for them. I did get some of their information into my stories, but I didn't see my job as doing their job. They wanted us to repeat night after night information on disease symptoms, etc. We have two minutes and fifteen seconds to do a story. We had the whole world [to cover] with SARS including Asia and Europe. If they [public health] want specific information disseminated, they should take out an ad in the newspaper.

I'm always jealous of the space newspapers get. They have more words to tell a story. The *Globe and Mail* is a very good newspaper. It has a lot of expertise in public health and medicine. Here at CBC, it was just me covering the scientific facts, the WHO travel advisory, and the economic impact—the print [media] did a more comprehensive job.

It was a challenge once the hospitals were shut down. We couldn't get any pictures, which is difficult for TV. It was hard to talk to the nurses who were sometimes not willing to talk in front of a camera and show their faces. There were cases in which nurses' children were shunned at daycare. It was rare, but it happened.

The public health officials had a daily news conference. We would all truck down to hear these four people talk to the media. No one knew who was in charge. We didn't have anyone like Dr. Julie Gerberding [CDC director] who comes across as a very strong leader. Our two government spokespersons were Dr. Colin D'Cunha and Dr. Jim Young, who was just a coroner. They were woefully inexperienced in infectious diseases, and our impression was that they had to be very careful, that government officials were leaning on them to not say too much. We got no science out of them. It was unsatisfactory.

We were hungry for basic science information, so we turned to our own experts. In the end, the politicians had to have them [our own science experts] on the podium. Even if they tried to have one spokesperson, we'd still get our own experts. Dr. [Donald] Low [microbiologist in chief, Mount Sinai Hospital, Toronto] was the most visible, but he had no power in government. He was willing to talk to the media and willing to say, "We don't know." It was refreshing to have someone willing to speak without fear of political fallout. There was political fallout for D'Cunha. He was eventually pushed out. They put in Sheela Basrur—she performed very well and had a calming effect. A lot of Canadians felt reassured. There was no panic here.

In my own reporting, I can't remember going to actual politicians to get their reaction to the WHO travel advisory and its economic repercussions. The political bureaucrats—Young and D'Cunha—gave us the same reaction as the politicians. We preferred to go to the scientists for their reaction and get a range of comments and opinions.

I think the media [eventually] became too caught up in SARS. We needed to take a step back. We reported only deaths, but a lot of people recovered. There were 450 cases and 33 deaths. SARS had a 10 percent mortality rate.

During SARS 2 [the second outbreak peak], the media were in denial. I admit I got too engaged after awhile. I just wanted it to be over with, and I let some of my reporting skills down. There's been criticism that the media hyped SARS, but I don't think that was the case in Toronto. It may have been true of the media elsewhere.

Communication could have been improved. The politicians should have backed off and let the scientists, the people who know what they are talking about, give the briefings. [This should happen even if] the buck stops with the politicians.[57]

CONCLUSION

Confusion develops during the initial stages of any public health crisis, such as a disease epidemic. People want to know what is going on—and journalists are among the first who need to know. They want to know about the medical and scientific aspects of the illness, who is leading the response to the crisis, and what efforts are being made to contain the outbreak. Depending on the nature of the crisis, those in charge may not know all the answers and may view the media with trepidation because of its potential power to misinform the public, and because of the potential harm that such misinformation can cause.

Officials might be reluctant to speak at the risk of saying something that could turn out to be inaccurate or misinterpreted. Journalists might interpret this caution as spin. Although admitting "I don't know" could be viewed by the media as honesty, government officials might view such statements as indicating failure or not being in control of the situation.

For example, during the anthrax crisis, Tommy Thompson went before the cameras in an attempt to reassure the public. Donald Henderson, who directed the WHO global smallpox eradication program, was one of the scientific experts advising Thompson:

> It was a reaction [providing false reassurances] that I have seen time and again by political leaders when, in fact, it is unclear as to what is happening. [Thompson] got a good deal of bad press because no one was quite sure what was happening, and that soon became apparent. It is important to have someone with professional knowledge, but often scientific experts are not good at communicating. They use technical terms that people don't understand. You have to have a known individual who is trusted and to whom the press is willing to turn. All too often, the press gets people in academia with no real knowledge of the practical aspects of crises.[58]

In 1947, Dr. Weinstein and his press staff handled media communications with great skill and success. They had advantages: a single spokesperson (Weinstein), credibility, public trust in government, and media support. But their success was not solely the result of preexisting advantages: they involved the press as partners in the dissemination of information and provided access to health officials who, in turn, provided prompt and accurate responses.

Of course, in 1947, much was known about smallpox. It was not a new disease or a bioterrorist attack, so health officials understood how to respond effectively. Furthermore, a vaccine was already available, and there was a public health and medical infrastructure in place to handle the crisis.

In the three later cases profiled, the disease outbreaks were surprises and caught government officials unaware. Anthrax was a bioterrorist attack, cryptosporidium was an unfamiliar water parasite, and SARS was a previously unknown virus for which there was no available treatment or vaccine.

It is not hard to understand, then, that the government officials in charge of responding to these crises had difficulty communicating with the media. Crisis and emergency risk communication strategies are meant to help leaders handle communication challenges during crises. All outbreaks come as surprises, however, and outbreaks of novel organisms, such as HIV/ AIDS and SARS, should be expected to continue for as long as human population pressures disrupt ecosystems.

Under these circumstances, crisis and emergency risk communication becomes even more important since so much uncertainty exists. For example, during a bioterrorist attack or an animal health crisis involving livestock, crisis and risk communication must be used not only by health officials, but also by law enforcement officials (in the case of a bioterrorist attack), and by agriculture officials (in the case of a livestock crisis). All of these officials must communicate with elected officials, with one another, and with the public about the known risks and how to minimize them. Their risk communication efforts must be coordinated, simple, and repetitive for everyone to understand.

Leaders must recognize that the media are neither foe nor docile ally. The press will choose its stories based on what it considers important, interesting, and timely. Although the press has changed since the mid-20th century, responsible journalists still report crises as accurately as possible. Government officials should also be aware that if they cannot provide the information that journalists seek, journalists will find experts who will. In such cases, the press may talk to alleged experts who are not knowledgeable at all.

Public health views the media as its key method of disseminating information to the general public. "The news media must be viewed as the conduit of information to the public and not as an afterthought," wrote Kay Golan, a former director of media relations for the CDC.[59] This type of partnership was illustrated by the 1947 smallpox outbreak in New York City.

However, the media might not view their role as the conduit of information for public health officials. For example, Maureen Taylor, the CBC television national health news reporter, didn't see her job as doing public health's job. She suggested that public health officials seek alternative means for getting their health information messages out.

The anthrax bioterrorist attacks in 2001 raised crisis risk communication challenges to a whole new level. Not only was it a public health crisis, but it involved a high-profile criminal investigation as well. No one knew that the spores could leak out of the envelopes and infect people. Public health officials, from the CDC to local health departments, did not know the answers to the most important scientific questions: who was at risk and what should be done to prevent infection in the different risk groups? Public health officials were unwilling to talk to the press.

Gursky, Inglesby, and O'Toole interviewed 37 public health officials, clinicians, government officials, journalists, and others directly involved in the anthrax attacks for a number of months after the crisis occurred.[60] They found that many public health officials did not consider media requests for information to be a priority and lacked media-savvy public affairs professionals. In addition, public health officials described tension between themselves and elected officials as to how much information should be released to the press.

In some cases, elected officials decided which groups of people should receive prophylactic antibiotics—occasionally, counter to state health officials' recommendations. The journalists reported considerable difficulty getting information from public health officials, who frequently ignored phone calls. Frustrated, journalists sought outside experts, scanned websites, and relied on unofficial contacts for information.[61]

Vicki Freimuth, director of communications at the CDC during the anthrax attacks, believes that much of what was reported about anthrax was inaccurate, because the spores used in the letter attacks were weaponized with characteristics different from those in the bacteria found in their natural state. Since little was known about weaponized anthrax, public health officials feared that acknowledging their ignorance would generate public panic—even though there were no data to support that assumption. As a result, many public health officials chose to not communicate with the media at all rather than acknowledge their lack of information.[62]

It was also difficult to select an appropriate spokesperson during the anthrax attacks. There were debates as to whether the spokesperson should be an elected official or a scientific expert. According to Freimuth, politicians make poor spokespersons during a crisis because they have a natural tendency to want to assert their control over the situation and to reassure the public. The public prefers honest and credible answers even if it is bad news. Public health leaders value scientific expertise over communication skills and frequently prefer not to be the primary spokespersons even though that is what the public wants.[63]

Freimuth wrote that the best-laid plans of the chain of command are frequently ignored during an actual crisis. Politicians want to be spokes-

persons but are not qualified, and public health officials are the most qualified but do not necessarily want the job. This conundrum frequently leads
to the inevitable question, "Who is in charge?"

During the anthrax crisis, public health officials used the Internet to disseminate information. The CDC posted transcripts from press briefings on
its Web site within hours after they were conducted. Unfortunately, the
information was not updated quickly enough to meet demand, and the system was overwhelmed.[64]

Newspaper advertisements, another form of public communication, were
used during the SARS outbreak in Toronto. Maureen Taylor, the Toronto
television news journalist who reported on SARS, suggested that newspaper advertisements would be a good strategy to get daily public health
information to the public. Not everyone shared this view, however.

"I think advertisements in newspapers would look biased and would
not be a good strategy [to disseminate information to the public]," said
Dr. Donald E. Low, microbiologist in chief, Mount Sinai Hospital, Toronto. "Our most effective strategy was to use the media to get the [public
health] message out."[65]

According to Dr. Richard Schabas, the chief of staff at York Central
Hospital, Richmond Hill, Ontario, one of the initial hospitals with SARS
cases, the newspaper advertisements were problematic:

> Just before Easter weekend, around April 19, when the initial SARS out-
> break was almost over, public health officials posted a full-page ad in the
> newspapers that said, "If you have any of these symptoms—headache, mal-
> aise, fever, or muscle aches—you should put yourself in quarantine." It was
> bizarre. If you look at it now, the people who put the ad out had no under-
> standing about what they were dealing with.[66]

Unlike the anthrax crisis in the United States, in which the question arose
as to who should serve as the spokesperson, in Canada, it was not necessarily who, but how many. The media and public health officials had different
opinions about the number of spokespersons needed during a press conference. The two journalists who covered the SARS outbreak in Toronto did
not consider a team of spokespersons an acceptable alternative to a single
leader. Both expressed frustration as to who was in charge.

"There should have been one spokesperson, but on the other hand, the
media wanted to hear from more than one person. I think that having more
than one spokesperson [at the press conferences] allowed the media to get
all the information they needed," said Low.[67] According to Schabas:

> I thought the media did a pretty good job reporting what was being told to
> them. The problem was that they were being told the wrong information.

Each day, there was a press conference that announced the latest deaths and the cumulative number of SARS cases. Presenting cumulative SARS cases is like announcing the day's rainfall based on the total rainfall for the year. The curve never goes down; it just keeps going up. This makes no sense, and what it did was create a picture of a large and growing outbreak that had no basis in reality. The outbreak had peaked by the third week of March and was petering out. What they should have done was present the new cases of SARS each day in order to put things into perspective. This is called the incidence rate and is taught the first day in basic epidemiology courses. The four horsemen[68] should have known better and should have presented to the press an epidemic curve so that people could follow exactly what was going on.[69]

Daniel Drache and Seth Feldman at York University in Toronto conducted a study on the media coverage of the 2003 SARS outbreak and found that the focus of the media changed as the epidemic evolved. Based on their analysis of more than 2,600 Canadian and American newspaper articles with SARS-related content over a 91-day period (March 16, 2003, to June 15, 2003), they determined that during the initial outbreak, the media focused almost exclusively on medical information about SARS and its management. As the epidemic continued, coverage increased on the political and economic aspects of the crisis.[70]

When the WHO travel advisory was announced on April 23, media coverage peaked even though the initial outbreak was essentially over.[71] The stories continued to focus more on the economic and political aspects of the epidemic, however, rather than on health. Furthermore, depending on their political leaning, newspapers criticized different aspects of government for their handling of the crisis. For example, the *National Post* criticized the federal government in Ottawa, whereas the *Toronto Star* focused its criticism on the provincial government of Ontario.[72]

Many interest groups, ranging from public health activists to private sector businesses and local and federal governments, see the media as a tool to send their messages. Some of these groups, such as public health activists and businesses, had conflicting objectives and messages. Public health tried to communicate that SARS was a grave threat, whereas the tourist industry, and Asian businesses in particular, sought to reassure the public that Toronto was safe. Caught between these conflicting interests, the media did not serve as a passive conduit for the stakeholders' messages but instead actively defined the crisis by deciding what to report.[73]

Griffin, Dunwoody, and Zabala found that in the 1993 cryptosporidium outbreak in Milwaukee, like the research on the Toronto SARS outbreak coverage, media coverage focused initially on the medical aspects of the illness, but it shifted with time to cover more newsworthy aspects of the story—such as how the parasite got into the water supply, the slow government response to complaints about water quality during the early days of the outbreak, and the delay between the outbreak and the boil water advisory.[74] The failure to communicate well had lasting implications: five months after the outbreak, almost 30 percent of Milwaukee residents still believed that their tap water was not safe to drink—and were less confident in their city government than before the outbreak.[75]

To assess the retrospective impact of the media messages on the public, five months after the cryptosporidium outbreak, the authors conducted a telephone survey of 610 adults who lived in an area served by the Milwaukee Water Works. They asked questions about their use of the media (newspapers, television, and radio) and personal worry about becoming ill from cryptosporidium in the future. They found a significant association between worries about one's own personal risk of getting the disease and attention to cryptosporidium information in newspapers, local television news, and radio media outlets. They found no significant difference among the three different media sources and level of worry, however. What did predict a greater concern about getting sick again was whether the individual had gotten sick during the outbreak or had stayed healthy.[76]

Accurate and effective communication can be a challenge even under the best circumstances. During a disease outbreak, the many risk concerns about the nature of the outbreak, such as who is at risk and who is in charge, combined with the conflicting, competing interests of various interest groups, make it easy for confusion to develop. For the media, epidemics represent opportunities for at least three types of stories: scientific/medical, political, and economic.[77] In the event of a bioterrorist attack, national security becomes a critical concern, and the criminal investigation generates additional interest.

Leaders who work with journalists to convey information to the public should do so with honesty and integrity. How an epidemic or bioterrorist attack is reported can change national and international perceptions and responses, even though the news might not reflect what is actually happening. The media should be responsible for the accuracy and integrity of what it reports, and ideally, the journalists covering disease crises should have expertise and knowledge in the subject area.

Clearly, the media does not serve as a passive conduit of information to the public. The media of the 21st century blends news, entertainment, and opinion 24 hours per day, 7 days per week. These conditions create challenges for all leaders to communicate effectively. Given the importance of public communication during a disease crisis, leaders should be required to have education, training, and practice in crisis and risk communication.

Chapter 9

ALL HANDS ON DECK

WORST CASE SCENARIOS

When public health crises or bioterrorist attacks impact normal societal functioning and overwhelm local capabilities, then political leaders need to declare a state of emergency and request assistance. The challenge during these scenarios is to have local, state, and federal officials work from the same script and interface with one another while working with others outside of government. The U.S. National Incident Management System established in 2003 facilitates communication and collaboration across many organizations and jurisdictions: emergency management, law enforcement, public health, hospitals, and others, all of which must work together in order to minimize loss of life.[1]

Political leaders, particularly at the local level, need to understand their roles and responsibilities and prepare for the worst case scenario. They need to reach out and develop relationships with local experts and know whom to turn to for help. They need to understand that there will be a critical period of time before state and federal assistance arrives, and their decisions could make the difference between many lives saved or lost. Poor political leadership can lead to disastrous outcomes such as the thousands of lives needlessly lost during Hurricane Katrina.

LEGAL CHALLENGES OF PUBLIC HEALTH AND BIOTERRORISM

Leaders need to be aware that legal challenges arise during public health crises—particularly bioterrorist attacks. The U.S. Constitution grants states the legal authority and responsibility for public health. State laws delineate state and local public health agencies' missions, functions, and powers. These laws are meant to safeguard individuals' rights by setting standards for actions, such as mass vaccination and quarantine policies during outbreaks.[2]

The problem is that public health laws vary from state to state, depending on each state's political and legal environments. Some legal experts consider these laws to be antiquated.[3] The 1988 Institute of Medicine report discussed in Chapter 1 recommended that states' public health laws be reformed.[4] In response to this challenge, in 1997, the Robert Wood Johnson and W.K. Kellogg foundations established "Turning Point," an initiative with the goal of improving public health across the United States. One of the products from this initiative was the Turning Point Model State Public Health Act, which is a comprehensive public health law meant to serve as a model for states to use to modernize and harmonize their public health laws, but it has raised concerns about the excessive powers it gives to public health officials over hospitals, physicians, and the public in the event of an infectious disease crisis.[5] A 2001 survey conducted by the Turning Point initiative suggests that relatively few states have passed statutes providing substantial public health reform.[6]

In addition to many states' outdated public health laws, the U.S. federal system of government was not designed to handle a bioterrorist attack. The division of responsibility between federal and state governments hinders response efforts: conflicting national security laws, criminal justice laws, state public health laws, and emergency response laws are all invoked. For example, a bioterrorist attack is an attack against the national security of the country, so it is a federal issue. At the same time, it is a public health crisis, so it is a state issue.[7] Under such circumstances, confusion is inevitable.

The United States has established policies that attempt to address potential confusion by defining the roles of federal and state agencies during terrorist attacks. When President Bill Clinton signed Presidential Decision Directive 39 in June 1995, the Department of Justice (DoJ) became the lead federal agency responsible for investigating and responding to terrorist attacks. The DoJ delegates the operational response to threats or acts of terrorism to the Federal Bureau of Investigation (FBI), and the Federal Emergency Management Agency (FEMA) supports the FBI while taking responsibility for incident management.[8]

The Department of Health and Human Services (HHS) and the Centers for Disease Control and Prevention (CDC) support state public health agencies. During the 2001 anthrax attacks, federal law enforcement and state public health officials struggled to work together.[9] A year later, the Association of State and Territorial Health Officials convened sessions with state health officials who had been involved in the bioterrorist attacks. Its primary recommendation for preparing for future attacks was for health officials to establish strong relations with high-ranking state law enforcement officials to avoid communication confusion. The association also noted that public health sometimes served as a communication bridge among federal, state, and local law enforcement officials who did not necessarily communicate well among themselves.[10]

Many local, state, and federal law enforcement officials worked in New Jersey during the anthrax crisis. James Collins was the Hamilton Township police chief during the crisis:

> There was never a situation in which they [the FBI] didn't share information with me. The FBI was the investigative agency in charge of determining who was responsible [for the anthrax attacks]. We were there to assist them. Our role as local law enforcement was to respond to suspicious packages with our HAZMAT (hazardous material) teams and to keep panic low.[11]

Kevin Hayden was commanding officer for the New Jersey State Police Office of Emergency Management during the 2001 anthrax crisis:

> In the state of New Jersey, the OEM [Office of Emergency Management] is part of the Division of State Police. Michigan is the only other state to have this arrangement. There are advantages [to this arrangement] including access to a lot of resources, structure, and discipline. The anthrax attack in the United States was a unique type of crime. Law enforcement in general did not have much experience in bioterrorism criminal investigation. We had a criminal investigation with a health issue [anthrax].
>
> The FBI in general was the lead agency for this type of investigation with support from the New Jersey State Police, local law enforcement, postal investigators, and the New Jersey Department of Health and Senior Services. The New Jersey State Police gave the FBI office space in our State Police Headquarters in Trenton. Kevin Donnovan was the FBI Special Agent in Charge (SAC) out of the Newark Office. He was the overall FBI lead. The New Jersey State Police assisted. The State Police, in cooperation with local law enforcement and county prosecutors, was also responsible for responding to thousands of anthrax scares, collecting specimens, and transporting them to the state health lab in Trenton. At the time, law enforcement had to develop threat criteria, evidence protocols, and just-in-time training for this type of response. In many cases, we had to rely on HAZMAT teams to collect samples.
>
> Dr. DiFerdinando [New Jersey State health commissioner] and Dr. Eddy Bresnitz [New Jersey state epidemiologist] did a great job in providing law enforcement with the health aspects of this type of exposure. They provided a lot of information that law enforcement would need. The postal authority actually tracked the letters and showed us how mail went through the postal machines.

> We got conflicting recommendations for treatment of anthrax exposure from federal [health] authorities. It was changing every day. They were influenced by public pressures and not medical decisions. It became a political issue.
>
> [Acting] Governor DiFrancesco and Attorney General John Farmer dealt with the political aspects of the crisis. They did a good job in that they let people do their jobs. There was no fighting by any of the agencies that we were involved with over who got in front of the cameras.[12]

Kenneth Shuey was part of the FBI investigation in New Jersey:

> I was the Senior Supervisory Special Agent in charge of the Trenton Resident Agency, Newark Division of the FBI. I was the on-scene commander and had meetings with public health. We had to learn about how anthrax affected people. . . . Dr. Eddy Bresnitz [the New Jersey state epidemiologist] was our main contact. The criminal investigation ran parallel to the public health investigation. Public health was our first concern and took precedence.[13]

By law, the FBI was in charge of the federal response to the anthrax crisis. Nevertheless, the individuals interviewed were cognizant of the fact that they were dealing with a public health crisis and stated that they made efforts to work collaboratively with New Jersey public health officials at the state level.

At the local level, there were few collaborative efforts between law enforcement and public health, aside from Mayor Glen Gilmore's sending police cars to pick up antibiotics for postal workers. Much of the local public health response was handled by the local private hospital.

A bioterrorist attack challenges the functioning of the U.S. federal system. As a national security threat, such a crisis requires a federal criminal investigation. In the case of the 2001 attacks, the FBI spent seven years investigating the crime and invented a new field, microbial forensics, in the process.[14] Federal law enforcement officials not only work with state and local law enforcement officials, they also have to interact with federal, state, and local public health officials.

At the same time, a bioterrorist attack is a state public health crisis requiring an epidemiologic investigation, medical treatment of the victims, medical screening of the potentially exposed, and mass vaccinations or prophylactic medications (if available) for those considered at risk. Since each state's public health infrastructure and capability is different, blending federal and state efforts across disciplines inevitably leads to complexity and confusion. Clarity of leadership and effective communication across the various government agencies are crucial.

IMPROVING PREPAREDNESS

One strategy to improve the collaboration between the federal government and the states is to equalize states' public health capabilities through federal quality improvement requirements. There have been efforts to do this through accreditation, but these efforts impose additional costs on an already cash-strapped public health field and are voluntary.[15]

A more realistic strategy might be to mandate infrastructures that facilitate better performance. For example, New Jersey's public health infrastructure is largely a local-level endeavor funded by local taxes, so the capabilities of each locality differ. In essence, it is a piecemeal system. In contrast, New York has full-service county health departments that receive funding from the state. The state mandates consistency across the localities, facilitating better biopreparedness planning.[16] However, different states have different needs, so what might work in one state might not work in another.

Another strategy would be to transform public health from a state to a federal responsibility. Currently, the CDC must be *invited* by states to investigate outbreaks. This arrangement is problematic because state public health departments and their epidemiological investigative capabilities vary considerably. Outbreaks such as the 1993 cryptosporidium crisis in Milwaukee, Wisconsin, are typically well underway by the time the CDC is invited to help.

The CDC could function more like other federal agencies (such as the Environmental Protection Agency [EPA] or the FBI), with field offices across the country that take charge of investigating outbreaks. The CDC has personnel posted in state and local health departments, although many of them are trainees who spend only two or three years in the field. In response to a directive from the secretary of HHS, the CDC developed the Career Epidemiology Officer program in 2003 to increase the number of epidemiologists trained in epidemic intelligence services (EIS) at the state and local levels.[17]

The CDC EIS officers are part of the Public Health Service (PHS) Commissioned Corps, which is one of the seven uniformed services in the United States. The Office of the Surgeon General manages the 6,000 full-time public health professionals in the PHS Commissioned Corps and deploys emergency response teams during public health crises such as the anthrax attacks.

Training and retaining qualified public health professionals, particularly epidemiologists, at the state and local level is difficult, however. In 2006, the Council of State and Territorial Epidemiologists (CSTE) found that most state health departments cited poor promotion opportunities and low salaries as major reasons for poor retention.[18] The CSTE estimates that the country needs about 1,200 more epidemiologists. In order to pay them, however, states are increasingly forced to rely on federal funding. In 2006, 75 percent of epidemiology funding came from the federal government.

In contrast, the FBI has its headquarters in Washington, D.C., and has 56 field offices in major U.S. cities and more than 400 resident agencies in smaller cities and towns.[19] Both law enforcement and environmental protection became federal responsibilities after policymakers recognized that criminal activity and air and water pollution cross state boundaries. Microbes, too, fail to recognize political borders.

A BETTER MODEL

The genesis of the EPA is a relevant model for a unified federal response to an epidemic or bioterrorist attack.[20] In the 1970s, public concern about the environment led President Richard Nixon to create the EPA through an executive order that combined 15 programs from three departments, two councils, and one commission into a single entity. In subsequent years, Congress passed environmental laws such as the Federal Environmental Pesticides Control Act and the Clean Air Act that the EPA implemented. In general, the EPA develops and enforces national environmental standards that states and tribal territories implement. The agency has 10 regional offices, laboratories, and research centers across the United States that conduct a number of surveillance activities, including measuring environmental radioactivity, evaluating emission control technologies, and assessing pesticide detection technologies in air and water, among other efforts.

If the EPA depended on state support, it would not have been able to achieve its successes. Likewise, innovative public health surveillance, research, and enforcement would be best accomplished at the federal level with federal mandates and support. If this approach were taken for public health, federal experts based in CDC field offices around the United States would handle multistate food-borne outbreaks, arthropod-borne disease outbreaks, multi-drug-resistant bacterial outbreaks, and bioterrorist attacks. This arrangement would allow the CDC to work with state and local public health partners to conduct proactive disease surveillance. It would also allow the CDC to work in tandem with the FBI as leaders when investigating the criminal and public health aspects of a bioterrorist attack.

EXPERTS' ADVICE

Two experts in public health were asked to discuss leadership at the national and state levels: Dr. Irwin Redlener, New York City, and Dr. Ruth Bekelman, Atlanta, Georgia.

Dr. Irwin Redlener, a physician and director of the National Center for Disaster Preparedness at Columbia University's Mailman School of Public Health and president of the Children's Health Fund, said:

Depending on the severity of the crisis, the president and the secretary of health and human services [HHS] would formally be in charge at the federal level with the CDC director reporting to the secretary. Yet, functionally, the director of the CDC would be making or recommending major strategies and priorities, but I'm not sure it would be so clean. If the past is any indication, there would be many competing voices, including authorities at every level of government and from a variety of agencies. The fact is that the crisis would be a situation in flux with many unanticipated issues coming up regularly, and experts would be falling all over themselves to be in front of the cameras. The reality is that on a technical or medical issue, there can be different ways of interpreting rapidly unfolding events, including who says what to whom. Overlap and confusion will likely prevail.

I think the situation might be helped by having an informed, empowered surgeon general as the person to whom the nation turns during a crisis. The surgeon general is in charge of the Commissioned Corps and has a smattering of other responsibilities at the moment. That position is often viewed, especially during the [George W.] Bush administration, as a political loose cannon. C. Everett Koop [a former surgeon general during the Reagan administration] was, in effect, a czar in leading a public health response to AIDS. He had a very public persona and was the embodiment of public health leadership. That is, in my mind, what would be needed in a major public health crisis.

Public health leadership is generally far from where it needs to be in some states; local officials are given a lot of independence. And in some of the nation's larger cities, such as New York and Los Angeles, federal disaster planning and response grants are received directly without flowing through state government.

In my view, I think there should be more federal control over the federal dollars that are provided to states and local governments, especially in planning for major public health emergencies. The fact is that congressional concern about terrorism has yielded a tremendous amount of federal funding to the table. But state and local officials have far too much latitude in what is done with and purchased by these federal disaster preparedness dollars without much accountability. We end up with a great deal of idiosyncratic spending, resulting in a random hodgepodge of readiness capabilities with far too much variance among communities in terms of what's been done with public resources.

Good, consistent leadership is essential for any large-scale public health program, particularly so with respect to disaster readiness. The American public has lost a great deal of confidence in our ability to prepare and respond. Good public health measures require that there is a credible messenger.

But now, the public health system is overstressed, underfunded, and losing credibility.

We need to be sure that we have strong, credible and empowered public health leaders if we are to have any hope of preparing properly and responding effectively to any major crisis.[21]

Dr. Ruth Berkelman is the Rollins Chair and director of the Center for Public Health Preparedness and Research at the Rollins School of Public Health at Emory University, Atlanta, Georgia. She was the deputy director of the National Center for Infectious Diseases (NCID) of the CDC from 1992 to 1997 and the assistant surgeon general from 1995 to 2000.

Who would be in charge is likely to depend on how disruptive a crisis is to normal societal function. If it becomes disruptive to society, then elected officials become more involved. At the state level, the governor is in charge, but the governor may decide to delegate some of the decision making. States vary in the strength of their public health leadership.

States have the authority to call the CDC for assistance. If a crisis crosses state lines, then federal involvement is more likely. The 1993 cryptosporidium outbreak in Milwaukee didn't cross state lines, although some patients were from other states. The CDC didn't play as major a role as in many other outbreaks. In addition, at the time, there was a scarcity of federal expertise on this emerging parasitic disease. The EPA [Environmental Protection Agency] didn't have expertise either.

The emergence of the Hantavirus was very different.[22] Some states saw a few previously healthy people die, but they didn't ask the CDC immediately for on-site assistance; they worked on the problem themselves with only limited laboratory assistance from the CDC. The IHS [Indian Health Service] called in the CDC through its own authority. Reservations are sovereign and not under state authority. After they requested assistance, the states also called for assistance.

Some states will invite the CDC in more readily than others. Some states would prefer to address outbreaks themselves and don't want the feds to come in. The state epidemiologist often calls the shots.

Public health is varied across jurisdictions. Some departments are highly competent and others less so. It is important to have some people medically trained to address the practicing physicians' and the public's concerns.[23]

PUBLIC HEALTH AND EMERGENCY MANAGEMENT

In an effort to coordinate the federal agencies in charge of protecting the United States, Congress passed the Homeland Security Act of 2002, which created the Department of Homeland Security (DHS), a new cabinet-level agency, and consolidated many executive branch agencies including

FEMA, the Animal and Plant Health Inspection Service (APHIS), and the U.S. Customs Service. On February 28, 2003, President George W. Bush issued Homeland Security Presidential Directive–5, which designated the secretary of homeland security as the principal federal official responsible for coordinating all federal responses to terrorist attacks.[24]

The directive also requires the secretary of DHS to develop and administer a National Incident Management System (NIMS)—guidelines to improve communication and collaboration among federal, state, local, and Native American tribal governments. These guidelines include an Incident Command System (ICS) in which leadership is given by either a single commander or team, depending on the magnitude of the disaster.[25]

WHO'S IN CHARGE?

Mark Ghilarducci is vice president and director of the Western States Regional Office of James Lee Witt Associates, a company that provides technical expertise and consultation services to government and the private sector on crisis and consequence management. He is the former deputy director of the Governor's Office of Emergency Services (under Governor Gray Davis) for the State of California, and he worked in the federal coordinating office with FEMA under President Bill Clinton:

> At the national level, the buck stops at the White House. The president appoints a federal coordinating officer (FCO) who is with FEMA and coordinates all federal agencies during a crisis response. The federal government is not set up to be the first responder. Instead, it is designed to support state government, which in turn supports the local governments. The federal government can and does provide additional resources that are critical to states and locals. In certain cases, such as a biohazard or a pandemic, you may need to shut down transportation, borders, and airports, so the federal government would take the lead [in these areas].
>
> During the Oklahoma City bombing, the FBI was the lead agency in charge of the crime scene. But it was also a disaster scene, so FEMA in support of state and local officials, coordinated the urban search and rescue operations. People who were trapped in the building had to be removed for emergency treatment or [if dead] recovered. The rescue and recovery operation needed to move forward, while the FBI needed to preserve evidence and concurrently move the investigation of the crime scene forward. This was an ongoing balancing act. Both disaster and crime scene operations had to be flexible and work together to achieve mutually agreed upon strategic objectives. At an agreed upon point when the rescue and recovery operations were complete, they [FEMA/Oklahoma City Fire] were able to turn the building over to the FBI so that its criminal investigation could be completed.

For tactical operations, most state and local and a few federal agencies use the ICS [Incident Command System], which incorporates a unified approach in which to build consensus. There is a hierarchy of decision making, and 99.9 percent of the time, leaders and commanders come to resolutions. Coordination is the cornerstone to any successful [response and recovery] operation. Without it, you get a situation like [Hurricane] Katrina.

[During a pandemic] HHS/CDC would be the lead federal agencies. FEMA would be in a support and coordination role. They would activate and coordinate the parameters of the National Response Framework[26] [previously known as the National Response Plan]. Local and state government emergency services, and the federal government as a whole, would be responding to this type of event. As such, NIMS and ICS would be utilized as they would in any incident management situation. In particular, this type of event would require extensive coordination and communication at every level of government and the private sector, as well as an extensive need for resources. NIMS and ICS would be critical for a comprehensive and coordinated response. This event may result in mayoral, gubernatorial, and presidential declarations of disaster, and FEMA would be instrumental in facilitating the disaster response and recovery as it would with any other type of disaster event.

The role of elected officials [mayors, county supervisors, governors] is to ensure competent emergency response/recovery staff and leadership. Elected officials need to keep the larger perspective of an evolving or urgent situation, provide policy oversight and leadership. They must maintain confidence with the public and show the public that they are in control of the situation. Given that every crisis situation will also be a political event to elected officials, how they respond to emergencies or disasters can make or break what responders are doing. It is critical to ensure that elected officials and emergency response/recovery staff understand each other's expectations and follow designated policies, procedures, and coordination systems.[27]

EPIDEMICS AND BIOTERRORIST ATTACKS: LEADERSHIP CHALLENGES

Epidemics and bioterrorist attacks are different from other natural or human-made disasters. Unlike bombings, fires, or hurricanes in which the events are finite and well defined, disease crises can develop slowly and insidiously over time. The beginnings of such crises are frequently missed. During the initial stages of an outbreak, people with nonspecific symptoms such as fevers, coughs, and chills seek medical care at their doctors' offices, clinics, or emergency rooms. They are usually sent home with symptomatic relief and told to return if symptoms worsen. During the anthrax attacks, physicians did not immediately diagnose the patients with the cutaneous form of the disease. Recognition that an attack had occurred did not happen until Dr. Larry Bush in Florida diagnosed the first case of inhalation anthrax.

Officials responsible for responding to disease crises should *assume* that diagnosis and reporting will be delayed. Leaders can be confronted with scientific uncertainty even when the crises are caused by naturally occurring agents. Trying to decide the best course of action might take time.

Disease crisis responses largely depend on robust public health, medical, and scientific infrastructures. With a severe epidemic, however, first responders such as fire, police, and EMT squads could have a role in medication distribution, law enforcement, and patient transport. Indeed, even postal workers have been recommended as resources to distribute medications to the general public during an anthrax attack.[28]

If a severe epidemic overwhelms the local public health and medical capabilities, in addition to help from the U.S. Public Health Service Commissioned Corps, state governors could call the National Guard and the military for public health or medical assistance.

PUBLIC HEALTH, THE MILITARY, AND THE NATIONAL GUARD

U.S. law allows the armed forces to provide humanitarian and civic assistance, including medical, surgical, dental, and veterinary care in foreign countries,[29] but the use of the military to provide aid within the United States is more complicated. In June 1878, Congress passed the *Posse Comitatus* Act to prevent local law enforcement officials in the post-Reconstruction South from conscripting army soldiers as police officers. This act has commonly been interpreted as prohibiting the armed forces from assisting law enforcement agencies, but this is not entirely accurate. The Coast Guard, for instance, is part of the Department of Homeland Security, and, as such, it is allowed to operate within the United States. Indeed, part of its mission is to protect the public in U.S. ports and waterways.

Nor does the act apply to the National Guard when it is operating in state-controlled status.[30] The National Guard has unique dual federal and state roles. In its federal role, the president can deploy it to serve in oversees conflicts or peacekeeping missions. In its state role, the governor can call it into action to respond to civil disturbances, earthquakes, fires, and storms.

The Robert T. Stafford Disaster Relief and Emergency Assistance Act (the Stafford Act) of 1988 circumvented some of the restrictions of the *Posse Comitatus* Act by allowing the president to provide Department of Defense (DoD) resources to any state in which the governor requests assistance during a major disaster.[31]

There are several examples of U.S. military assistance within the United States. In 1992, the response to Hurricane Andrew in South Florida included more than 22,000 troops deployed for disaster assistance. After the Northridge, California, earthquake of 1995, almost 800 troops were deployed. In April 1995, almost 400 federal military forces were sent to assist state and local officials after the Murrah Federal Building bombing in Oklahoma.[32] During the 2005 Hurricane Katrina disaster along the Gulf Coast, more than 50,000 National Guard and 20,000 active military personnel were deployed to assist in the response.[33] Although no federal troops were deployed during the 2001 anthrax crisis, the U.S. Army Medical Research Institute for Infectious Disease provided expert laboratory testing of thousands of anthrax specimens.[34]

As noted earlier, Homeland Security Presidential Directive–5 (HSPD-5) designated the secretary of DHS as the principal federal official responsible for coordinating all federal response operations for all major disasters and for developing a National Response Framework. The framework defines 15 Emergency Support Functions (ESF) annexes (supplementary documents to the National Response Framework core document). These ESF annexes facilitate coordinated disaster responses by specifying the federal agency that is in charge of areas such as transportation, emergency management, public health, and agriculture. In all of the ESF annexes, the DoD serves in a supportive role.[35]

For example, the secretary of HHS is in charge of ESF #8, which coordinates federal public health, medical, and veterinary medical assistance to state, local, and tribal authorities.[36] The HHS may request DoD support for patient treatment, disease surveillance, laboratory diagnostics, and evacuation.[37]

For epidemics involving veterinary diseases, ESF #11 places the secretary of the U.S. Department of Agriculture (USDA) in charge. If an epidemic involves a zoonotic agent that can infect both animals and humans, then the USDA and the HHS work together. The Department of the Interior is in charge of wildlife epidemics. The DoD could be called in to provide transportation, laboratory, and veterinary support. If an animal health crisis such as foot-and-mouth disease were to occur in the United States, then the U.S. Army Corps of Engineers would be summoned to provide logistical expertise and resources for mass slaughter and carcass removal.[38]

Joseph M. Palma, MD, MPH, a colonel in the U.S. Air Force and former acting deputy assistant to the Secretary of Defense for chemical/biological defense, describes the military's interaction with the states during times of crisis:

> The primary mission of the DoD is to fight the nation's wars. The DoD is not chartered for planning for epidemic management, but it is clearly aware

of its backup capability. We don't actively plan to be the first responders, although we do have the capabilities to support disasters if called upon.

After 9/11, the United States established the Northern Command [NORTHCOM].[39] Although forces are assigned during times of emergencies, such as disaster relief operations, no forces are currently assigned. Its role is to serve as a military support vehicle to coordinate with states and Canada [and Mexico] during a national emergency. The chairman of the Joint Chiefs allocates forces as needed during deliberate planning.

The different branches of the military have different missions. I can't see [that] the air force would be enlisted to provide ground forces, but I do see where it would be essential to move things by airlifting. The army and marines provide ground troops, and they do each have medical departments to support local needs if called upon.[40]

The U.S. Army Medical Command (MEDCOM) has medical facilities across the United States, Europe, and Japan. MEDCOM has 27,000 soldiers and 20,000 medical soldiers in field units. More than 30,000 medical soldiers are in the Army Reserve and the National Guard.[41]

The navy has two hospital ships: the *Comfort* and the *Mercy*. Both are 1,000-bed hospital facilities with 12 fully equipped operating rooms, laboratories, radiological capabilities, pharmacies, and helicopter decks. They can be fully activated in five days. The *Mercy* is based in San Diego, California, and the *Comfort* is stationed in Baltimore, Maryland.[42]

U.S. military assistance has not been limited to domestic disasters. On April 5, 1991, the United Nations (UN) Security Council provided the justification for international humanitarian or human rights interventions with Resolution 688—passed in response to the repression of the Kurdish population in Northern Iraq.[43] Since then, a number of disasters have required international assistance from both government and nongovernment organizations.

On December 26, 2004, a magnitude 9 (Richter scale) earthquake off the coast of Indonesia resulted in repetitive massive tsunami waves that killed more than 220,000 people around the Indian Ocean rim. Humanitarian teams from many nations responded, including the U.S. DoD. Their missions were to assess the situation and prioritize interventions, help the victims, and prevent additional morbidity and mortality.

One of the challenges in international disasters is for external humanitarian teams *not* to take over, but to assist local communities and indigenous regional and national agencies to reestablish their self-sufficiency. Another challenge is to establish good working relationships between the military and civilian teams. Both military and civilian organizations provide unique areas of expertise necessary for disaster response. The military brings logistical expertise and resources such as vehicles and helicopters for transportation and supply deliveries of water, food, and tents. The military can also provide security, a critical necessity that nongovernmental agencies cannot do in times of crisis. Civilian-military discord may arise when the different leaders insist on being in charge, do not coordinate efforts, or compete for public support and recognition. Nongovernmental organizations and UN personnel expect that the line between military and civilian humanitarian activities will not be blurred.[44]

Military personnel must walk a fine line providing their material and logistical resources without exacerbating their image as agents of the strategic interests of their respective governments. In addition, they must provide the aid in an impartial way, particularly in areas experiencing civil discord. Regardless of these challenges, the military has much to offer in humanitarian assistance.[45]

Forty-eight hours after the Indonesia earthquake, the U.S. National Command Authority authorized the commander of the U.S. Pacific Command to call up Joint Task Force 536. Joint Task Force 536 sent a forward element to the Royal Thai Navy Air Base in Utaphao, Thailand; it was joined by the III Marine Expeditionary Force command element from Okinawa, Japan. On January 3, 2005, the two elements were designated as Combined Support Force (CSF) 536. In addition, the USS *Abraham Lincoln* medical team provided preliminary assessments of the disaster areas: hundreds of thousands of people had been killed, more were homeless and separated from families, and many roads were impassable.[46]

A command coordination center (CCC) was set up at CSF 536 headquarters in Utaphao and served as the site where military and civilian efforts were coordinated. The UN, World Health Organization (WHO), World Food Programme (WFP), and many nongovernmental organizations sent liaisons to CCC daily meetings and provided field updates. The military provided its rapid response and communications capabilities, logistical expertise, and early medical forensics support.[47]

In addition to the immediate impact of the tsunami, there was concern that infectious disease outbreaks would develop from a lack of clean water and sanitation. That threat was largely averted because of the coordinated international efforts. The DoD's Naval Medical Research Unit in Jakarta served as a reference laboratory for disease surveillance and prevention.[48] This laboratory is one of five DoD laboratories stationed around the world to conduct research and surveillance of influenza and other emerging infectious diseases.[49]

Named the Global Emerging Infections Surveillance and Response System (DOD-GEIS), these research facilities were established in response to Presidential Decision Directive NSTC-7, issued in 1996 by President Clinton. The directive expanded the DoD mission to include global emerging infectious disease research, surveillance, training, and response.[50]

Headquartered in Silver Spring, Maryland, DOD-GEIS consists of five overseas laboratories based in Jakarta, Indonesia; Lima, Peru; Cairo, Egypt; Bangkok, Thailand; and Nairobi, Kenya, and two domestic laboratories in San Diego, California, and San Antonio, Texas.[51]

These laboratories have provided important services in outbreak investigations, disease surveillance, and vaccine development. From October 2005 to February 2006, they responded to 66 outbreaks in 22 countries. In collaboration with the CDC, WHO, host country governments, and other organizations, the laboratories identified a number of diseases, including avian influenza A (H5N1) in Indonesia, Iraq, Egypt, Turkey, and Kazakhstan.[52]

In March 2006, the DoD-GEIS laboratories received $39.28 million for avian and pandemic influenza surveillance activities. One year later, the Institute of Medicine issued an evaluation of the DoD-GEIS Influenza Program. It found that the program was effectively managed and executed, and it made a number of recommendations, including that the laboratories expand their public health mission, conduct more surveillance of animal populations, work more closely with host country laboratories, and coordinate with domestic partners and host countries in planning pandemic influenza responses.[53]

In summary, the military has extensive expertise in logistics, material and laboratory support, research, and rapid response capabilities. It would likely be summoned to respond to severe public health and animal health crises that overwhelm state and local capabilities. The military's challenge would be to work with civilian agencies to rebuild local capabilities while devising an exit strategy.

CONCLUSION

In the United States, a response to a severe, societal-disrupting disease outbreak would involve many leaders across federal, state, and local agencies. The challenge, under such circumstances, is that as the severity of the crisis increases, the complexity of the response necessarily increases as well. A complex response adds to the risk for inefficiency and confusion. Although the secretary of DHS would serve as the coordinator for major disasters, and DHS developed guidelines such as the National Incident Management System to facilitate communication and collaboration among agencies and jurisdictions, inherent legal and infrastructure weaknesses in the federal system could still hinder response efforts.

Bioterrorism highlights these inherent weaknesses. A bioterrorist attack is an attack against a nation's national security (a federal responsibility), and at the same time, it is a public health crisis (a state responsibility in the

United States). Unfortunately, public health in the United States is a rather piecemeal affair: states vary widely in their public health laws, infrastructures, capabilities, and, as Dr. Redlener noted, how they spend federal disaster preparedness funds. Dr. Berkelman pointed out that the CDC must be invited by states to investigate an outbreak, and that some states are more inclined than others to ask the federal agency for assistance. This arrangement means that outbreaks are typically well underway by the time CDC is summoned. Such inefficiencies do not bode well when time is of the essence.

One strategy to address this problem would be to federalize public health. Just as pollution and criminals do not recognize political borders, neither do microbes. Making public health a federal responsibility would provide federal resources, establish field offices in states and major cities, and potentially reduce the disparities among states' capabilities. The structure and functioning of the EPA provide a model that could be adapted for public health.

If state and local capabilities were completely overwhelmed by a severe disease outbreak, such as pandemic influenza or a bioterrorist attack, then the governor would have to request federal assistance from FEMA, the National Guard, the U.S. Public Health Service, and even the military. However, state and local elected officials need to understand that the arrival of federal assistance takes time, and if many states and localities were affected and federal resources were stretched thin, then they might still be on their own. How state and local elected officials prepare for such worse case scenarios could make the difference between life and death for many people.

Chapter 10

CONCLUSION

This book has explored leadership during disease crises. Its goal was to understand why leadership problems develop by examining five disease crises using newspaper articles, books, government inquiries, and medical literature. Many of the leaders who participated in these crises were interviewed, including elected officials, public health professionals, physicians, veterinarians, scientists, journalists, and law enforcement officials.

At least two leaders emerge in a crisis: the elected official and the appointed professional bureaucrat. In severe crises, there likely would be many more leaders from various agencies involved, potentially complicating the chain of command and increasing the risk for miscommunication or disputes. In some cases, particularly at the local, municipal, or county level, a public health professional might not be in place to recommend major interventions such as mass vaccinations, prophylactic antibiotic distribution, or quarantine. In these circumstances, the elected official would have to serve in both leadership capacities.

The disease crises and interviews revealed four key themes that address leadership problems. First, engaged, informed, and prepared elected officials are absolutely critical for preventing leadership problems. They are, after all, ultimately in charge and responsible for all decisions. Elected officials must have established relationships with key players, including appointed officials and nongovernmental professionals, based on mutual respect and trust. They must have strong communication skills, be willing to listen to others' opinions, and know how much decision-making authority they want to delegate to their appointees during a crisis. Relationships between appointed officials and nongovernmental professionals are just as important as those between elected and appointed officials.

Second, when scientific information is lacking, elected officials occasionally need to rely on their common sense and best judgment when making crisis response decisions. All crises begin with some level of chaos and confusion. However, when a crisis involves a new disease, involves animals such as livestock, or involves a bioterrorist attack, decision making becomes particularly difficult because the scientific advice might be inadequate.

Third, political and bureaucratic officials must be effective communicators with each other and with the media. Both elected officials and professional appointees must communicate early and often with the media to show the public that they are working hard to address the crisis. The leaders serve different, but equally important, roles. The media prefer to get scientific information from appointed professionals and scientific experts and political information from the elected officials. When leaders give false reassurances that everything is under control when, in fact, it is not, they risk losing their credibility.

Fourth, a nation's legal frameworks and organizational infrastructures can influence decision making. For example, a bioterrorist attack in the United States is a federal responsibility because it is an attack against national security. At the same time, it is a public health crisis and as such is a state responsibility. This duality of responsibility can create inherent leadership confusion.

CRITICAL NEED: PREPARED ELECTED OFFICIALS

Misunderstandings or poorly developed relationships between elected officials and professional bureaucratic appointees can lead to poor response outcomes. Two models of political leadership during a crisis were presented: the Giuliani model and the Glendening model. In the Giuliani model, the elected official makes the key decisions with expert advice from appointees and scientific advisors. In the Glendening model, the appointee makes the key decisions with scientific advice from experts and political support from the elected official. Either of these models can be successful as long as the participants understand and accept their roles.

Elected officials are ultimately responsible for crisis response outcomes. They decide how much or how little decision-making authority they will delegate. In the United States, the personality of the elected official largely determines which model is used. In parliamentary systems such as those in the UK and Canada, the Glendening model appears to prevail unless a specific problem develops necessitating that the elected official take command.

The designers of the tabletop exercises "Dark Winter"[1] and "TOPOFF" mentioned in chapter 1 assumed that the senior elected officials would follow the Giuliani model and not delegate decision-making authority to their professional appointees but, rather, make their own decisions based on advice from scientific experts. As the crises described in this book illustrate, this situation is not necessarily the case. Many of the elected officials preferred to delegate decision making.

During the 2001 anthrax crisis, New Jersey Acting Health Commissioner George DiFerdinando did not have an understanding of his relationship with New Jersey Acting Governor Donald DiFrancesco. DiFrancesco delegated decision making to DiFerdinando, who made decisions without political backup and ran into difficulties with the Centers for Disease Control and Prevention (CDC) and the mayor of Hamilton Township over closing the Hamilton postal facility, taking nasal swabs, and distributing prophylactic antibiotics to postal workers. In contrast, Drs. Georges Benjamin, secretary of health in Maryland, and New York City Health Commissioner Neil Cohen understood their relationships with their respective elected officials and acted accordingly. Maryland Governor Parris Glendening provided political support and delegated decision-making authority to Benjamin during the crisis (the Glendening model). New York City Mayor Rudolph Giuliani largely kept his decision-making authority and preferred to get expert advice from Cohen and others (the Giuliani model). Regardless of the model used, the elected official should listen to others' opinions.

In some crises, elected officials delegate decision making to their appointees but subsequently have to reassume decision-making responsibilities when conflicts develop. During the 1993 cryptosporidium outbreak in Milwaukee, Wisconsin, Mayor John Norquist had to assume decision-making duties when mediating a dispute between the health commissioner and the water works secretary. They could not agree on a boil water advisory. The mayor's office originally considered the crisis a public health issue and wanted the health commissioner to be the point person in an effort to avoid making the response look politically motivated. However, the dispute forced the mayor to issue a boil water advisory himself.

It is the responsibility of the elected official to establish an understanding with his or her appointee early in the administration as to the nature of their relationship during a crisis. Even if the relationship evolves with time, the professional appointee should not have to guess how much or how little decision-making authority he or she would be delegated in the event of a crisis. Elected officials without appointees should assume that they will be making all decisions and be responsible for crisis response planning and execution.

This was the case with Mayor Glen Gilmore during the anthrax crisis in New Jersey. The infrastructure was lacking: there was no local- or county-level public health official with whom he could establish a relationship and give decision-making responsibilities. Fortunately, he had the foresight to establish a relationship with the local hospital administrator *before* the crisis hit. He had also identified where to get antibiotics beforehand, so he was prepared. Elected officials who do not do their homework of identifying key players and resources before a crisis will likely find themselves scrambling to catch up as the critical hours of opportunity fade away.

RELATIONSHIPS BETWEEN LEADERS

During the foot-and-mouth disease (FMD) crisis in France, Dr. Isabelle Chmitelin attributed much of the government's success at containing the disease to the good relationship she had with the director of food safety, who, in turn, was well connected with the minister of agriculture and provided him with information. The minister had to be convinced that FMD was important and that it required rapid decisions even though it did not infect humans.

Relationships built on respect and trust matter not only between elected officials and their appointees but also between public health and health care professionals. For example, in Florida, Drs. Larry Bush and Jean Malecki knew and trusted each other after serving on committees together. Bush knew to call her when he suspected anthrax in his patient. The process of disease identification and reporting occurred rapidly and smoothly. In contrast, Dr. Daksh Patel did not know whom to contact in New Jersey and subsequently did not contact anybody. Eventually, people from the federal government interviewed him. He assumed they were from the military. This situation was less than optimal.

Agriculture officials need to have good relationships with veterinarians, farmers, and others in the agriculture industry. During the British FMD crisis, the veterinarians and farmers, among others, protested against the government's controversial slaughter policies. Among the many things that went wrong during the crisis, the lack of leadership, consensus, and cooperation was a significant factor.

WHEN SCIENCE DOES NOT HAVE THE ANSWERS

Leaders sometimes must rely on their common sense and best judgment when making decisions involving a new disease, a disease in animals, or a bioterrorist attack. Elected officials without a scientific or technical background might be reluctant to make such difficult decisions and either do not make them or wait until experts give them advice. If they do decide to seek expert advice, they should have the best scientific experts available, and be willing to listen to them. The decision-making process needs to be open and honest (transparent) in order to gain public trust. However, even with expert scientific advice, decisions can be difficult. There might be little or no scientific information available, and advisors might disagree with one another.

A significant problem during the FMD crisis was the conflict between the mathematical modelers and the virologists who served as scientific advisors. After David King, the UK's chief scientific advisor, heard Nick Brown's false reassurances, he formed an ad hoc group of mathematical modelers to study the outbreak. They recommended the controversial 24/48-hour slaughter policy. Drs. Paul Kitching and Alex Donaldson, veterinarian virology experts, disagreed with the modelers' recommendations.

Kitching went on television news and announced that the mathematical models used to predict the spread of the virus were based on parameters from the 1967 FMD outbreak. The 1967 virus spread much more readily than the 2001 virus, he said, so the drastic slaughter policies were unnecessary. This conflict between the experts confused the policymakers, the media, and the public.

Even without disagreements between scientific advisors, decisions can be difficult, as they were during the decade-long bovine spongiform encephalopathy (BSE) crisis in the UK. Political leaders sought expert scientific advice regarding the risks to humans. The science experts initially assumed that the disease would behave like scrapie, which did not affect humans, but they advised that potentially dangerous animal products be kept from baby food just in case the disease could affect humans.

Lord John MacGregor, the minister of MAFF (Ministry of Agriculture, Fisheries and Food), used his common sense and decided that potentially dangerous animal products should be kept from all human food products regardless of the age of the consumer. That decision proved prescient, since years later scientists proved that the BSE agent could affect humans. Unfortunately, for the 143 people afflicted with vCJD (a variant of Creutzfeldt-Jakob disease), it was too late.

Similarly, New Jersey Health Commissioner DiFerdinando used his medical knowledge, judgment, and common sense to recommend that all postal workers from the Hamilton mail distribution facility receive prophylactic antibiotics. Scientific evidence was not available to support the notion that anthrax spores could leak out of envelopes, but he did not want to take any chances. The CDC officials disagreed with him and refused to provide antibiotics from the national stockpile.

To address these issues, Jean-Claude Manuguerra recommended that expert advisory committees be long-standing and not assembled in a rapid fashion during a crisis. Such an advisory committee should be multidis-ciplinary so that various expert points of view are heard when addressing novel infectious disease and bioterrorist agents. Members of long-standing committees know and trust one another and should feel more comfortable admitting what they know and do not know than would members of hastily assembled committees. These advisory committees should provide advice, but they should not make decisions or serve as substitutes for leaders. As Dr. David Sencer stated, leadership by committee means there is no lead-ership. Only elected officials or their designated appointees should make decisions.

The avian influenza outbreak in Asia created daunting leadership dilem-mas. Whenever a novel disease impacts livestock, such as avian influenza or BSE, the risk that it can spread to humans is a serious concern, since many new diseases do emerge from animals and infect humans. The lead-ers of the Hong Kong avian influenza outbreak had their decision made for them: the farmers demanded that their poultry be slaughtered, and the government reimbursed them for their losses since demand for poultry plummeted in the wake of the crisis.

Political leaders in Indonesia faced avian influenza and decided *not* to make any decisions but instead ignored the threat. In this example, the po-litical leaders deferred to political pressure from agricultural industry lead-ers who did not want their livelihoods threatened. This example highlights the importance of getting the support of the affected industry (and that of the public) for tough policy decisions. The national director of animal health and the health minister made recommendations that were ignored. As a result of these poor decisions and inactions, Indonesia has had more cases of human avian influenza than any other nation.

THE PUBLIC COMMUNICATION ROLES
OF DIFFERENT LEADERS

Poor communication skills or inaccurate communications can lead to confusion. Elected officials want to be in front of the cameras, but some have a tendency to provide false reassurances. The media want informa-tion from the professionals and scientists who understand the nature of the disease crisis. These individuals are not necessarily effective public communicators. The end result can be leadership confusion and poor credibility.

During the anthrax crisis, U.S. Secretary of Health and Human Services Tommy Thompson gave false reassurances to the media that the anthrax death in Florida was due to a naturally occurring exposure. Thompson was criticized for providing false information and for assuming the role that should have been filled by a physician. Dr. Jeffrey Koplan, the director of the CDC, on the other hand, very rarely appeared before the cameras during the entire crisis.[2]

During the 2001 FMD crisis in the UK, both Nick Brown, the minister of MAFF, and Jim Scudamore, the chief veterinarian, provided false reassurances that the crisis was under control. As the crisis worsened, they lost credibility and were subsequently removed from decision-making authority. The turnover in leadership, as well as the conflict between the scientific advisors, created distractions from the crisis response and cost precious time and effort. Tony Blair, the prime minister, ultimately took over.

Communication errors occurred during the BSE crisis when MAFF officials falsely reassured consumers that British meat was safe to eat. Risk communication skills, such as admitting what is known and not known, are especially important when scientific uncertainty clouds a crisis. In the case of the BSE crisis, the disease-causing agent was novel, and it was unknown whether it could affect humans. Eventually, after it was discovered that the prion could affect humans, the officials lost their credibility and public outrage ensued.

Communication problems can arise if there are too many scientific and medical experts in front of the cameras. For example, during the 2003 SARS crisis in Toronto, Canada, leadership confusion arose because too many experts and public health officials were talking to the media. Andre Picard, the public health reporter for the *Globe and Mail,* referred to the four physician leaders as "the four physicians of the apocalypse." He thought that there should have been one principal messenger.

Two of the physician spokespersons were the Ontario commissioners of public health and public safety. According to Donald Low, these two commissioners were equally in charge but reported to different elected officials. The commissioners gave conflicting views and opinions which worsened the leadership confusion.

The Canadian elected officials did not appear before the cameras until after the World Health Organization (WHO) issued a travel advisory against Toronto. Mel Lastman, the mayor of Toronto, was so poorly informed about the outbreak that he worsened public confidence with his ignorant statements. Fortunately, Case Ootes, the deputy mayor, was available to substitute for him. The media faulted the elected officials at all levels of government for poor political leadership.

The Canadian SARS crisis illustrates that even if elected officials delegate decision making to their professional appointees, they still need to demonstrate political leadership by communicating early and often with the media. Behind the scenes political support is important, but the public wants to know that their elected officials are actively engaged in the crisis response.

The 1947 smallpox outbreak in New York City has been hailed as a gold standard in crisis communications even though more people died from vaccine adverse reactions than from the disease itself.[3] In this outbreak, Mayor William O'Dwyer provided political support and delegated decision making authority to Dr. Israel Weinstein, the commissioner of health. Weinstein was the primary spokesperson to the media although the mayor publicly showed his support for Weinstein's actions. Weinstein maintained a simple and clear message and had a good relationship with the media.

Although the media want to see and hear from elected officials, they prefer a single, credible individual with scientific expertise to serve as an official spokesperson during a crisis. Unfortunately, public communication skills are generally not taught in schools of medicine, veterinary medicine, or public health. Many public health professionals, physicians, veterinarians, and scientists lack the skills needed to communicate to the public during a crisis.

Public communication is taught in leadership institutes, but it should be part of the curriculum in all schools of medicine, veterinary medicine, and public health. Understanding how the 21st-century media works is crucial for all individuals who might find themselves answering questions in front of cameras and microphones during a crisis. News coverage is changing as newspapers downsize, television news loses its audience, and the Internet becomes an increasing force in disseminating information.[4]

During the 2009 swine flu crisis, the Internet and social networking services such as Facebook and Twitter played major roles in disseminating information. The media of the 21st century blends news and entertainment that can result in misinformation. The initial death rates reported in Mexico were high, and Mexican leaders made difficult but appropriate decisions to close schools, museums, sporting events, and other social venues. Unfortunately, the global media generated continuous stories about the new flu killer that contributed to over-reactions and poor policy decisions by government officials in many countries.

Approximately six weeks after the new flu virus was first reported, health officials discovered that it wasn't as deadly as initially thought. The media soon lost interest and coverage dropped markedly except for the day that WHO declared a global pandemic. This crisis illustrates that government officials, the media, and Internet social networking services share the responsibility of providing accurate information, not speculation or exaggeration, about a developing epidemic. Just as leaders should avoid giving false reassurances, they should also avoid embellishing unsubstantiated or preliminary information since hysteria can lead to inappropriate decisions, needless suffering, and harm.[5]

LEGAL AND ORGANIZATIONAL STRUCTURES AND CRISIS LEADERSHIP

Leadership and decision making are influenced by a country's legal framework and infrastructure. For example, the U.S. federal system of government creates a legal conundrum when dealing with a bioterrorist attack. A bioterrorist attack is an attack against U.S. national security, so it is a federal responsibility. The FBI is the lead federal agency. At the same time, it is a public health crisis, so it is a state responsibility.

The CDC is not the lead agency, but it serves a supportive and advisory role to the state health departments, when it is called in. Some states will invite the CDC in to investigate an outbreak more readily than others. Since microbes do not recognize arbitrary political borders, and states' public health capabilities vary, this organizational infrastructure is inefficient and hinders decision making. In addition, if an outbreak does not cross state lines, then CDC involvement is less likely. For example, the 1993 cryptosporidium outbreak in Milwaukee, Wisconsin, was almost over by the time state and local officials identified the crisis and called the CDC for help.

This legal framework guarantees that federal outbreak investigations and leadership are delayed. Instead, if public health were a federal responsibility, the CDC would be the lead agency, analogous to the FBI's role in law enforcement, in responding to bioterrorist attacks.

In addition to the disparities across state and local health departments, current public health laws hinder the CDC and FBI from working together in parallel leadership positions. Since the FBI is the lead agency when responding to bioterrorist attacks, it has seasoned agents distributed across the country. In contrast, CDC officials at the state and local level are primarily trainees. During the anthrax crisis, the CDC was stretched thin because it had to send many different teams to different states. According to DiFerdinando, the CDC sent a less experienced team to New Jersey that wound up hindering rather than facilitating an appropriate response. If public health were a federal responsibility, then experienced CDC personnel would be stationed around the country, decreasing the risk of being stretched too thin during a crisis. This arrangement would also facilitate the CDC's working with state and local public health partners in conducting proactive disease surveillance and research.

In the event of severe, societal-altering epidemics or bioterrorist attacks, federal, state, and local emergency management, the U.S. Public Health

Service, FEMA, the National Guard, and the military would likely be summoned to assist in the government response. In the case of deadly zoonotic diseases such as avian influenza infecting livestock and humans, an important response policy would be to slaughter the animals in an attempt to curtail disease spread. Agriculture and health officials would have to communicate, collaborate, and coordinate when responding to these events.

In some cases, the military would have to be called in to supply logistical expertise and personnel. The British FMD crisis illustrated the important role of the military in handling crises involving livestock. Military personnel were needed for the slaughter and disposal of millions of animals.

In the United States, Homeland Security Presidential Directive–5 designates the secretary of the Department of Homeland Security as the lead federal official in charge of coordinating all federal efforts in response to terrorist, including bioterrorist, attacks. The directive also requires the implementation of the National Incident Management System, a set of guidelines that includes the Incident Command System, which is a standardized all-hazard framework designed to reduce the risk of miscommunication and poor chain of command among leaders of different response agencies.

Problems can occur if elected officials do not mediate disputes between leaders of different agencies since only elected officials have the legal authority to make final policy decisions. It was Mayor Norquist who settled the dispute between two different agency leaders during the 1993 cryptosporidium crisis.

TRAINING ELECTED OFFICIALS

Given how critical elected officials' roles and responsibilities are during crises, one would expect that elected officials would consider participating in training exercises a priority. Frank Keating, governor of Oklahoma, and other elected officials participated in "Dark Winter," but Bill Owens, the governor of Colorado, did not participate in the TOPOFF exercise described in chapter 1. Keating, who had taken office shortly before the Oklahoma City bombing in April 1995, might have been more cognizant of the importance of preparedness than was Owens, who did not have such experience.[6] Owens's primary experience with disaster during his tenure as governor occurred two years after TOPOFF: in 2002, he was criticized by Colorado business owners and the tourist industry for his comment that "all of Colorado was burning" when eight major wildfires engulfed the state.[7]

It is unknown how many elected officials have participated in tabletop exercises or leadership-training seminars to prepare them for severe disease crises.[8] However, in recognition of the need to educate local leaders on emergency preparedness and response, the U.S. Department of Homeland Security awarded a three-year $1.9 million grant in September 2007 to the National League of Cities (NLC) to deliver 40 one-and-a half-day training programs across the country to elected and appointed officials. The course is meant to cover all emergencies, including epidemics, and how local elected and appointed officials need to be part of the planning and response processes. On March 14, 2009, the first of four pilot programs was offered in Washington, D.C. Fifty-six elected and appointed officials from around the nation attended. This course is an important beginning in preparing leaders for future disease crises.[9]

Crises involving microbes present unique challenges. Ideally, all elected officials and public health and agriculture officials would possess political, communication, management, and organizational skills that would enable them to respond to outbreaks quickly and effectively. Regardless of whether elected officials prefer to make their own decisions based on expert advice or delegate decision making to professional appointees, they must recognize that their political leadership is crucial for any effective response. They must also be willing to give credit, when credit is due, to those whom they gave decision-making responsibilities. The media, in whatever form, should be viewed as an important partner in disseminating information to the public, because ultimately, the media and public will decide whether the government's response is a failure or a success.

NOTES

CHAPTER 1: UNDERSTANDING LEADERSHIP

1. M. H. Spooner, "Disease in Animals, Suicide in Humans," *Canadian Medical Association Journal* 169 (2003): 329.

2. L. H. Kahn and J. A. Barondess, "Preparing for Disaster: Response Matrices in the USA and UK," *Journal of Urban Health* 85 (2008): 910–22.

3. Institute of Medicine, *The Smallpox Vaccination Program: Public Health in an Age of Terrorism* (Washington, DC: National Academy of Sciences, 2005), 26.

4. Centers for Disease Control and Prevention, "Smallpox Fact Sheet: Smallpox Disease Overview," February 6, 2007. http://www.bt.cdc.gov/agent/smallpox/overview/disease-facts.asp.

5. Centers for Disease Control and Prevention, "Update: Adverse Events Following Smallpox Vaccination—United States," *Morbidity and Mortality Weekly Report* 52 (2003): 278–82. http://www.cdc.gov/mmwr/preview/mmwrhtml/mm5213a4.htm.

6. D. J. Kuhles and D. M. Ackman, "The Federal Smallpox Vaccination Program: Where Do We Go From Here?" *Health Affairs* Suppl. July–December 2003. Web Exclusives: W3–503–10. http://content.healthaffairs.org/cgi/content/full/hlthaff.w3.503v1/DC1.

7. Institute of Medicine, *The Future of Public Health* (Washington DC: National Academy Press, 1988), 4: 77–90.

8. Ibid.

9. Ibid.

10. Ibid.

11. L. H. Kahn, "A Prescription for Change: The Need for Qualified Physician Leadership in Public Health," *Health Affairs* 22 (2003): 241–48.

12. IOM, *The Future of Public Health,* 4.

13. Ibid., 127–32.

14. Ibid., 13–15, 119.

15. IOM, *The Future of the Public's Health in the 21st Century* (Washington DC: National Academies Press, 2003).

16. Ibid, 120–22.

17. K. Umble, D. Steffen, J. Porter, et al., "The National Public Health Leadership Institute: Evaluation of a Team-Based Approach to Developing Collaborative Public Health Leaders," *American Journal of Public Health* 95 (2005): 641–44.

18. Trust for America's Health, "Ready or Not 2008?" http://healthyamericans.org/reports/bioterror08/.

19. Ibid.

20. T. O'Toole, M. Mair, and T.V. Inglesby, "Shining Light on 'Dark Winter'," *Clinical Infectious Diseases* 34 (2002): 972–83.

21. The Dark Winter scenario has been criticized for choosing an extreme model for the spread of smallpox. See M. Enserink, "How Devastating Would a Smallpox Attack Really Be?" *Science* 296 (2002): 1592–95.

22. T. Inglesby, R. Grossman, and T. O'Toole, "A Plague on Your City: Observations from TOPOFF," *Clinical Infectious Diseases* 32 (2001): 436–45.

23. Ibid.

24. M. Weber, "Politics as a Vocation," in *From Max Weber: Essays in Sociology,* trans. and ed. H.H. Gerth and C. Wright Mills (New York: Oxford University Press, 1946/1958), 77–128.

25. R. Pear, "Embattled Disease Agency Chief Is Quitting," *New York Times,* February 22, 2002.

26. J. Bennet, "The Bush Years: C.E.O., U.S.A." *New York Times,* January 14, 2001.

27. Pear, "Embattled Disease Agency Chief Is Quitting."

28. E.N. Suleiman, "Introduction," in *Bureaucrats and Policy Making. A Comparative Overview,* ed. E.N. Suleiman (New York: Holmes and Meier, 1984), 3–7.

29. P. Krugman, "Find the Brownie," Op Ed., *New York Times,* September 26, 2005.

30. E.N. Suleiman, "From Right to Left. Bureaucracy and Politics in France," in *Bureaucrats and Policy Making,* 107–35.

31. R. Rose, "The Political Status of Higher Civil Servants in Britain," in *Bureaucrats and Policy Making,* 136–73.

32. Ibid.

33. J.M. Burns, *Leadership* (New York: Harper & Row, 1978), 1–3.

34. Ibid, 15–28.

35. Ibid., 302.

36. B. Kellerman, "Leadership as a Political Act," in *Leadership: Multidisciplinary Perspectives,* ed. E.N. Suleiman (Englewood Cliffs, NJ: Prentice Hall, 1984), 63–89.

37. M.A. Hill, "The Law of the Father. Leadership and Symbolic Authority in Psychoanalysis," in *Leadership: Multidisciplinary Perspectives,* 23–38.

CHAPTER 2: THE LONG MARCH TO IMPROVING THE PUBLIC'S HEALTH

1. J. Duffy, *The Sanitarians. A History of Public Health* (Chicago: University of Illinois Press, 1990), 35–65.

2. Ibid.

3. Smallpox, yellow fever, and influenza are caused by viruses. Plague and cholera are caused by bacteria. Viruses are pieces of genetic material that infect the host's cells. They are unable to replicate by themselves and are technically not alive. Antibiotics do not work against viruses. Bacteria consume nutrients and reproduce themselves. They are alive, and there is even evidence that they communicate with one another. Antibiotics will kill or stun bacteria, although many are developing resistance to these drugs.

4. M. Wheelis, "Biological Warfare at the 1346 Siege of Caffa," *Emerging Infectious Diseases* 8 (2002): 971–75. http://www.cdc.gov/ncidod/eid/vol8no9/01-0536.htm.

5. W. H. McNeill, *Plagues and Peoples* (New York: Random House, 1977).

6. K. B. Patterson and T. Runge, "Smallpox and the Native American," *American Journal of Medical Science* 323 (2002): 216–22.

7. J. B. Tucker, *Scourge. The Once and Future Threat of Smallpox* (New York: Grove Press, 2001), 20–22. See also Wheelis, "Biological Warfare."

8. The term *outbreak* is often used interchangeably with *epidemic*. *Outbreak* means a sudden increase, or eruption, such as an outbreak of measles. Sometimes, *outbreak* is used to denote a geographically limited epidemic, for example, in a school or a town. *Epidemic* is the preferred scientific term, but the words will be used synonymously in this book. A *pandemic* is an epidemic on a continental or global scale. For example, HIV/AIDS is a global pandemic.

9. McNeill, *Plagues and Peoples.*

10. Ibid.

11. C. De Paolo, *Epidemic Disease and Human Understanding. A Historical Analysis of Scientific and Other Writings* (Jefferson, NC: McFarland and Company, 2006). See also L. I. Conrad, "Epidemic Disease in Formal and Popular Thought in Early Islamic Society," in *Epidemics and Ideas* ed. T. Ranger and P. Slack (Cambridge, England: Cambridge University Press, 1992), 77–99.

12. Duffy, *The Sanitarians,* 5–8.

13. G. Rosen, *A History of Public Health* (New York: MD Publications, 1958), 6–21.

14. Duffy, *The Sanitarians,* 5–8.

15. De Paolo, *Epidemic Disease and Human Understanding.*

16. Rosen, *A History of Public Health,* 87–102.

17. Ibid.

18. G. Dinc and Y. I. Ulman, "The Introduction of Variolation 'A La Turca' to the West by Lady Mary Montagu and Turkey's Contribution to This," *Vaccine* 25 (2007): 4261–65.

19. Ibid.

20. Ibid.

21. A.J. Morgan and S. Parker, "Translational Mini-Review Series on Vaccines: The Edward Jenner Museum and the History of Vaccination," *Clinical and Experimental Immunology* 147 (2007): 389–94. See also N. Barquet and P. Domingo, "Smallpox: The Triumph over the Most Terrible of the Ministers of Death," *Annals of Internal Medicine* 127 (1997): 635–42; and D.R. Hopkins, *Princes and Peasants. Smallpox in History* (Chicago: University of Chicago Press, 1983), 77.

22. E.Y. Bridson, "Iatrogenic Epidemics of Puerperal Fever in the 18th and 19th Centuries," *British Journal of Biomedical Science* 53 (1999): 134–39.

23. C. Hallett, "The Attempt to Understand Puerperal Fever in the Eighteenth and Nineteenth Centuries: The Influence of Inflammation Theory," *Medical History* 49 (2005): 1–28.

24. Bridson, "Iatrogenic Epidemics of Puerperal Fever."

25. J. Duffy, *A History of Public Health in New York City 1625–1866* (New York: Russell Sage Foundation, 1968), 101–23.

26. Ibid.

27. Duffy, *The Sanitarians,* 35–65.

28. Ibid.

29. Ibid., 66–92.

30. A.F. La Berge, *Mission and Method. The Early Nineteenth-Century French Public Health Movement* (Cambridge, England: Cambridge University Press, 1992): 14–20.

31. W. Coleman, *Death Is a Social Disease. Public Health and Political Economy in Early Industrial France* (Madison: University of Wisconsin Press, 1982), 4–33.

32. La Berge, *Mission and Method,* 14–20, 24–33.

33. Rosen, *A History of Public Health.*

34. Unknown, "Introduction," in E. Chadwick, *On an Inquiry into the Sanitary Condition of the Labouring Population of Great Britain* (Edinburgh, Scotland: University Press, 1965), 1–7, 149, 236. See also La Berge, *Mission and Method*: 14–20, 291–300.

35. G. Gill, S. Burrell, and J. Brown, "Fear and Frustration—The Liverpool Cholera Riots of 1832," *The Lancet* 358 (2001): 233–37.

36. S. Burrell and G. Gill, "The Liverpool Cholera Epidemic of 1832 and Anatomical Dissection—Medical Mistrust and Civil Unrest," *Journal of the History of Medicine and Allied Sciences* 60 (2005): 478–98.

37. Rosen, *A History of Public Health.* Chadwick's report cited the work of Villermé as well as the work of other French hygienists, including Jean-Baptiste Parent-Duchâtelet.

38. C-E.A. Winslow, *The Conquest of Epidemic Disease. A Chapter in the History of Ideas* (Princeton, NJ: Princeton University Press, 1943), 271–76.

39. P.V. Johansen, H. Brody, N. Paneth, S. Rachman, and M. Rip, *Cholera, Chloroform, and the Science of Medicine. A Life of John Snow* (New York: Oxford University Press, 2003), 4–13.

40. W.H. Frost, "Introduction," in *Snow on Cholera 1813–1858* (New York: Oxford University Press, 1936), xx.

41. P.V. Johansen, H. Brody, N. Paneth, S. Rachman, and M. Rip, *Cholera, Chloroform, and the Science of Medicine. A Life of John Snow* (New York: Oxford University Press, 2003), 39–41.

42. H. Brody, M.R. Rip, P. Vinten-Johansen et al., "Map-Making and Myth-Making in Broad Street: The London Cholera Epidemic, 1854," *The Lancet* 356 (2000): 64–68. See also S.W.B. Newsom, "Pioneers in Infection Control: John Snow, Henry Whitehead, the Broad Street Pump, and the Beginnings of Geographical Epidemiology," *Journal of Hospital Infection* 64 (2006): 210–16; and Winslow, *The Conquest of Epidemic Disease,* 271–79.

43. Newsom, "Pioneers in Infection Control."

44. Duffy, *The Sanitarians,* 93–109.

45. Ibid.

46. Ibid.

47. P.M. Dunn, "Oliver Wendell Holmes (1809–1894) and His Essay on Puerperal Fever," *Archives of Disease in Childhood—Fetal & Neonatal Edition* 92 (2007): F325–F327.

48. T.D. Noakes, J. Borresen, T. Hew-Butler et al., "Semmelweis and the Aetiology of Puerperal Sepsis 160 Years on: An Historical Review," *Epidemiology and Infection,* June 7, 2007: 1–9.

49. I. Semmelweis, *The Etiology, Concept, and Prophylaxis of Childbed Fever,* trans. and ed. Carter K. Codell, (Madison: University of Wisconsin Press, 1983), 63–113.

50. Ibid.

51. Bridson, "Iatrogenic Epidemics of Puerperal Fever."

52. Noakes et al., "Semmelweis and the Aetiology of Puerperal Sepsis."

53. R. Dubos, *Louis Pasteur Free Lance of Science* (New York: Da Capo Press, 1950), 220–30.

54. Ibid., 244–46.

55. B.L. Ligon, "Robert Koch: Nobel Laureate and Controversial Figure in Tuberculin Research," *Seminars in Pediatric Infectious Diseases* 13 (2002): 289–99.

56. R. Munch, "Review: On the Shoulders of Giants. Robert Koch," *Microbes and Infection* 5 (2003): 69–74.

57. Ligon, "Robert Koch."

58. J.S. Sartin, "Infectious Diseases During the Civil War: The Triumph of the 'Third Army,'" *Clinical Infectious Diseases* 16 (1993): 580–84.

59. I.M. Rutkow, *Bleeding Blue and Gray. Civil War Surgery and the Evolution of American Medicine* (New York: Random House, 2005), 66–81. See also E. Fee and T.M. Brown, "The Unfulfilled Promise of Public Health: Déjà vu All Over Again. We Have Not Learned the Lessons of Our Public Health History," *Health Affairs* 21 (2002): 31–43.

60. Rutkow, *Bleeding Blue and Gray.*

61. Ibid.

62. Ibid., 82–114.

63. Sartin, "Infectious Diseases During the Civil War."

64. Rutkow, *Bleeding Blue and Gray,* 324.

65. Rosen, *A History of Public Health,* 200–69; Fee and Brown, "The Unfulfilled Promise of Public Health."

66. Mullen, *Plagues and Politics*: 17. See also U.S. Department of Health and Human Services. Office of the Surgeon General. http://www.surgeongeneral.gov/aboutoffice.html#historysg.

67. Mullen, *Plagues and Politics,* 20–30.

68. Duffy, *The Sanitarians,* 126–37.

69. Ibid., 138–56.

70. Ibid.

71. C-E.A. Winslow, *The Life of Hermann M. Biggs* (Philadelphia: Lea & Febiger, 1929), 91–100.

72. Ibid., 39, 69–74.

73. Ibid., 107–15.

74. Pan American Health Organization, *Pro Salute Novi Mundi. A History of the Pan American Health Organization.* Pan American Health Organization publication, 1992, 18–25.

75. Ibid.

76. Ibid.

77. H. Markel, *Quarantine! East European Jewish Immigrants and the New York City Epidemics of 1892* (Baltimore, MD: Johns Hopkins University Press, 1997), 5.

78. Mullen, *Plagues and Politics,* 32–57.

79. Ibid., 35–40, 111. Surgeon General John B. Hamilton opened the Hygienic Laboratory in 1887 in a room at the Marine Hospital on Staten Island. The laboratory eventually moved to Washington, D.C., and became the National Institutes of Health.

80. J. M. Barry, *The Great Influenza,* (New York: Penguin Books, 2004), 308–13.

81. Ibid., 310–14.

82. Ibid., 178–79.

83. H. Markel, A. M. Stern, J. A. Navarro et al., "Nonpharmaceutical Influenza Mitigation Strategies, U.S. Communities, 1918–1920 Pandemic," *Emerging Infectious Diseases* 12 (2006): 1961–64.

84. N. P. Johnson and J. Mueller, "Updating the Accounts: Global Mortality of the 1918–1920 'Spanish' Influenza Pandemic," *Bulletin History of Medicine* 76 (2002): 105–15.

85. Ibid.

86. Mullen, *Plagues and Politics,* 86–104.

87. Yakima Health District history. http://www.co.yakima.wa.us/Health/info/about_us.htm.

88. Mullen, *Plagues and Politics,* 86–104.

89. Ibid., 26–40.

90. Ibid.

91. Ibid., 104–27.

92. Ibid., 99, 104–27.

93. D.S. Wei, "Szeming Sze, MD. Obituary," *Journal of the American Medical Association,* 281 (1999): 579. See also S. Sze, *The Origins of the World Health Organization: A Personal Memoir, 1945–1948* (Boca Raton, FL: LISZ, 1982).

94. Sze, *The Origins of the World Health Organization,* 1–10.

95. Ibid., 17–20.

96. A. Bokazhanova and G.W. Rutherford, "The Epidemiology of HIV and AIDS in the World," *Collegium Antropologicum* 30 (2006, Suppl. 2): 3–10. See also F. Gao, E. Bailes, D.L. Robertson et al., "Origin of HIV-1 in the Chimpanzee *Pan troglodytes troglodytes,*" *Nature* 397 (1999): 436–41; and M. Peeters, V. Courgnaud, B. Abela et al., "Risk to Human Health from a Plethora of Simian Immunodeficiency Viruses in Primate Bushmeat," *Emerging Infectious Diseases* 8 (2002): 451–57.

97. United Nations General Assembly Special Session, "Resolution adopted by the General Assembly. Declaration of Commitment on HIV/AIDS," August 2, 2001. http://www.un.org/ga/aids/coverage/FinalDeclarationHIVAIDS.html.

98. L.K. Altman, "Leaving Platform That Elevated AIDS Fight," *New York Times,* December 30, 2008.

99. H. Burkhalter, "The Politics of AIDS: Engaging Conservative Activists," *Foreign Affairs* 83 (2004): 8–13.

100. M. Spector, "Annals of Science. The Denialists," *The New Yorker,* March 12, 2007: 31–38.

101. National Library of Medicine, "The C. Everett Koop Papers. Biographical Information." http://profiles.nlm.nih.gov/QQ/Views/Exhibit/narrative/biographical.html.

102. United Nations Press Release, "World Population Will Increase by 2.5 Billion by 2050." http://www.un.org/News/Press/docs//2007/pop952.doc.htm.

103. World Health Organization, "2005 International Health Regulations." http://www.who.int/csr/ihr/en/.

104. K.E. Jones, N.G. Patel, M.A. Levy et al., "Global Trends in Emerging Infectious Diseases," *Nature* 451 (2008): 990–94.

CHAPTER 3: MICROBES AS WEAPONS

1. S.H. Harris, *Factories of Death. Japanese Biological Warfare 1932–45 and the American Cover-Up* (London: Routledge, 1994), 75–112.

2. R.A. Etzel, "Mycotoxins," *Journal of the American Medical Association,* 287 (2002): 425–27. (A mycotoxin is a fungal toxin.)

3. J.K. Smart, "History of Chemical and Biological Warfare: An American Perspective" in *Textbook of Military Medicine,* eds., F.R. Sidell, E.T. Takafuji, and D.R. Franz (Washington, DC: Office of the Surgeon General, Borden Institute, 1997), 9–13.

4. M. Wheelis, "Biological Warfare Before 1914," in *Biological and Toxin Weapons: Research, Development and Use from the Middle Ages to 1945,* ed. E. Geissler and J.E. van Courtland Moon (Oxford, UK: Oxford University Press, 1999), 13–15.

5. Ibid., 21–25.

6. M. Wheelis, "Biological sabotage in World War I," in *Biological and Toxin Weapons: Research, Development and Use from the Middle Ages to 1945,* ed. E. Geissler and J. E. van Courtland Moon (Oxford: Oxford University Press, 1999), 35–62.

7. J. Witcover, *Sabotage at Black Tom. Imperial Germany's Secret War in America, 1914–1917* (Chapel Hill, NC: Algonquin Books, 1989). Bombing within in the United States is described in R. L. Koenig, *The Fourth Horseman. One Man's Secret Mission to Wage the Great War in America* (New York: Perseus Books Group, 2006), 83–116.

8. Koenig, *The Fourth Horseman,* 86–90, 280–81.

9. S. H. Harris, *Factories of Death. Japanese Biological Warfare 1932–45 and the American Cover-Up* (London: Routledge, 1994), 18–30.

10. S. H. Harris, "The Japanese biological warfare programme: an overview," in *Biological and Toxin Weapons: Research, Development and Use from the Middle Ages to 1945,* eds., Erhard Geissler and John Ellis van Courtland Moon, *SIPRI Chemical & Biological Warfare Studies* no. 18 (Oxford: Oxford University Press, 1999), 127–152.

11. E. Regis, *The Biology of Doom. The History of America's Secret Germ Warfare Project* (New York: Henry Holt, 1999), 9–21.

12. In 1932, 100 yen equaled about $28. So 200,000 yen equaled about $56,000. See H. T. Patrick, "The Economic Muddle of the 1920s," in *Dilemmas of Growth in Prewar Japan,* ed. J. W. Morley (Princeton, NJ: Princeton University Press, 1971), 233. In 2008 dollars, the amount would be approximately $826,607 using the Dollar Times inflation calculator. (http://www.dollartimes.com/calculators/inflation.htm).

13. Harris, *Factories of Death,* 18–32.

14. Ibid., 18–38.

15. Ibid., 30–45, 75–88.

16. Ibid., 43–50.

17. Global Security, "Weapons of Mass Destruction (WMD) Biological Weapons Program." http://www.globalsecurity.org/wmd/world/japan/bw.htm.

18. L. A. Cole, *Clouds of Secrecy. The Army's Germ Warfare Tests over Populated Areas* (Savage, MD: Rowman and Littlefield, 1990), 12–20; and Harris, *Factories of Death,* 203.

19. Harris, *Factories of Death,* 203–207. See also E. Regis, *The Biology of Doom. The History of America's Secret Germ Warfare Project* (New York: Henry Holt and Company, 1999), 9–21.

20. Smart, "History of Chemical and Biological Warfare," in *Medical Aspects,* 42–47.

21. Ibid.

22. L. A. Cole, *Clouds of Secrecy. The Army's Germ Warfare Tests over Populated Areas* (Savage, MD: Rowman and Littlefield, 1990), 12–20.

23. Ibid., 75–104.

24. Sarin and VX are liquid chemical warfare agents. They work either through direct contact with eyes or on skin or through the inhalation of vapors. Small amounts can be lethal.

25. Smart, "History of Chemical and Biological Warfare," 62–63.

26. The Biological and Toxin Weapons Convention Website. http://www.opbw.org/.

27. K. Alibek and S. Handelman, *Biohazard. The Chilling True Story of the Largest Covert Biological Weapons Program in the World—Told from the Inside by the Man Who Ran It* (New York: Random House, 1999), 40–44.

28. Tularemia (also called Rabbit Fever) is a bacterial disease of rabbits that can infect people. Marburg viruses are deadly hemorrhagic fever viruses such as Ebola, which can cause people to bleed to death.

29. J. Cirincione, J. B. Wolfsthal, and M. Rajkumar, *Deadly Arsenals. Nuclear, Biological, and Chemical Threat,* 2nd ed. (Washington DC: Carnegie Endowment for International Peace, 2005), 57–68. See also J. Miller, S. Engelberg, and W. Broad, *Germs. Biological Weapons and America's Secret War* (New York: Simon & Shuster, 2001), 165–68; and Alibek and Handelman, *Biohazard,* 137–47.

30. Miller, Engelberg, and Broad, *Germs,* 15–33.

31. Ibid.

32. D. E. Kaplan and A, Marshall, "The Cult at the End of the World," *Wired Magazine,* July 1996, Issue 4.07. http://www.wired.com/wired/archive/4.07/aum.html.

33. Miller, Engelberg, and Broad, *Germs*, 151–64.

34. Kaplan and Marshall, "The Cult at the End of the World."

35. Ibid.

36. Ibid.

37. K. B. Olson, "Aum Shinrikyo: Once and Future Threat?" *Emerging Infectious Diseases* 5 (1999): 513–16. http://www.cdc.gov/ncidod/EID/vol5no4/olson.htm.

38. S. Shane, "Portrait of Anthrax Suspect's Troubled Life," *New York Times,* January 3, 2009. http://www.nytimes.com/2009/01/04/us/04anthrax.html.

39. R. J. Jackson, A. J. Ramsay, C. D. Christensen et al., "Expression of Mouse Interleukin-4 by a Recombinant Ectromelia Virus Suppresses Cytolytic Lymphocytic Responses and Overcomes Genetic Resistance to Mousepox," *Journal of Virology* 75 (2001): 1205–10.

40. J. Cello, A. V. Paul, and E. Wimmer, "Chemical Synthesis of Poliovirus cDNA: Generation of Infectious Virus in the Absence of Natural Template," *Science Online,* 2002. http://www.sciencemag.org/cgi/content/full/297/5583/1016.

41. National Research Council, *Biotechnology Research in an Age of Terrorism* (Washington, DC: National Academies Press, 2004).

42. NSABB draft report. http://www.biosecurityboard.gov/NSABB%20 Draft%20DUR%20Ov%20Framewk8%20for%20public%20posting%20 041907%20mtg2.pdf.

CHAPTER 4: RISING TO THE OCCASION

1. L. J. Marcus, B. C. Dorn, and J. M. Henderson, "Meta-Leadership and National Emergency Preparedness: A Model to Build Government Connectivity," *Biosecurity and Bioterrorism* 4 (2006): 128–34.

2. L. H. Kahn and J. A. Barondess, "Preparing for Disaster: Response Matrices in the USA and UK," *Journal of Urban Health* 85 (2008): 910–22.

3. C. M. Greene, J. Reefhuis, and C. Tan, "Epidemiologic Investigations of Bioterrorism-Related Anthrax, New Jersey 2001," *Emerging Infectious Diseases* 8 (2002). http://www.cdc.gov/ncidod/EID/vol8no10/02-0329.htm. See also, C. G. Tan, H. S. Sandhu, D. C. Crawford, et al., "Surveillance for Anthrax Cases Associated with Contaminated Letters, New Jersey, Delaware, and Pennsylvania, 2001," *Emerging Infectious Diseases* 8 (2002). http://www.cdc.gov/ncidod/EID/vol8no10/02-0322.htm.

4. L. M. Bush, B. H. Abrams, A. Beall et al., "Index Case of Fatal Inhalational Anthrax Due to Bioterrorism in the United States," *New England Journal of Medicine* 345 (2001): 1607–10.

5. L. A. Cole, *The Anthrax Letters. A Medical Detective Story* (Washington, DC: Joseph Henry Press, 2003).

6. Ibid.

7. D. B. Jernigan, P. L. Raghunathan, B. P. Bell et al., "Investigation of Bioterrorism-Related Anthrax, United States, 2001: Epidemiologic Findings," *Emerging Infectious Diseases* [serial online] 8 (2002). http://www.cdc.gov/ncidod/EID/vol8no10/02-0353.htm.

8. M. W. Thompson, *The Killer Strain. Anthrax and a Government Exposed* (New York: HarperCollins, 2003).

9. Greene, Reehuis, Tan et al., "Epidemiologic Investigations of Bioterrorism-Related Anthrax, New Jersey, 2001."

10. Ibid.

11. Thompson, *The Killer Strain,* 114–16.

12. George T. DiFerdinando Jr. (MD, MPH; Co-Director New Jersey Center for Public Health Preparedness at University of Medicine and Dentistry of New Jersey (UMDNJ; former acting Commissioner of Health, NJDHSS), telephone interview, June 10, 2004.

13. United States Census 2002 Population Estimate. http://quickfacts.census.gov/qfd/states/34/34021.html.

14. M. Winerip, "Our Towns; Hail the Mayor (Whose Name Isn't Giuliani)," *New York Times,* November 14, 2001, p. 14.

15. E. Ramsey, "Hoping to Ease Hamilton Tax Burden, Mayor Gilmore Eyes Business Growth," *Mercer Business,* August 1, 2001. http://findarticles.com/p/articles/mi_qa3697/is_200108/ai_n8954302/.

16. The governor at the time was acting Governor Donald DiFrancesco, who took over when Christine Todd Whitman left to head the U.S Environmental Protection Agency.

17. Mayor Glen D. Gilmore, personal interview, December 21, 2006.

18. W. R. MacKenzie, N. J. Hoxie, M. E. Proctor et al., "A Massive Outbreak in Milwaukee of Cryptosporidium Infection Transmitted Through the Public Water Supply," *New England Journal of Medicine* 331 (1994): 161–67. Turbidity (cloudiness) of water is used as a proxy for bioload (microbiologic contamination).

19. *The Milwaukee Journal,* "Callers Boil at Excuses for Bad Water," April 14, 1993.

20. *The Milwaukee Journal,* "Water Works Failed to Tell Health Office About Complaints," April 14, 1993.

21. D. Behm, "Water Crisis Was Over Before It Began," *The Milwaukee Journal,* May 2, 1993.

22. *Capital Times,* "Unraveling Water Mystery Takes Some Super Sleuthing," April 12, 1993.

23. M. Marchione, "Doctor Solves Crucial Part of Illness Puzzle," *The Milwaukee Journal,* April 8, 1993.

24. L. H. Kahn, "A Prescription for Change: The Need for Qualified Physician Leadership in Public Health," *Health Affairs* 22 (2003): 241–48.

25. T. Cuprisin, "A Longer View of a Very Long Week of Water Crisis," *The Milwaukee Journal,* April 11, 1993.

26. Editorial, "Public Deserves Full Accounting," *The Milwaukee Journal,* April 9, 1993.

27. J. Manning, "Norquist Wants Fines for Barnyard Runoff," *Milwaukee Sentinel,* April 9, 1993.

28. *The Milwaukee Journal,* "Health Official Apologizes for Cryptosporidium Comments," December 7, 1993.

29. *The Milwaukee Journal,* "Chvala Blames Governor for Weakness of Water Law," April 13, 1993.

30. C. Gilbert, "Mayor Earns Praise, Faces More Questions," *The Milwaukee Journal,* April 18, 1993.

31. MacKenzie, Hoxie, Proctor et al., "A Massive Outbreak." See also W. Koch, "Milwaukee's Nightmare. Scores Die from Illnesses Linked to Contaminated Water," *Houston Chronicle,* October 3, 1996.

32. M. H. Kramer, B. L. Herwaldt, R. L. Calderon et al., "Surveillance for Waterborne-Disease Outbreaks States, 1993–1994," *Morbidity and Mortality Weekly Report,* 45 (1996): 1–33. http://www.cdc.gov/mmwr/preview/mmwrhtml/0004081 8.htm.

33. M. Kissinger, "Scandal Tests Norquist's Mettle," *Milwaukee Journal Sentinel,* January 13, 2001. http://www3.jsonline.com / news / metro / jan01 / norq14011 301a.asp?format=prin.

34. John Norquist (former Mayor of Milwaukee), telephone interview, January 28, 2007.

35. John Norquist, telephone Interview, January 12, 2007.

36. N. S. Zhong, B. J. Zheng, Y. M. Li et al., "Epidemiology and Cause of Severe Acute Respiratory Syndrome (SARS) in Guangdong, People's Republic of China, in February, 2003," *The Lancet* 362 (2003): 1353–58.

37. Ibid.

38. WHO, "Consensus Document on the Epidemiology of Severe Acute Respiratory Syndrome (SARS)." http://www.who.int/csr/sars/en/WHOconsensus.pdf.

39. M. Pottinger, A. Regalado, and M. Cohen, "Officials Alarmed by Spread of Respiratory Illness," *Wall Street Journal,* March 17, 2003, A3.

40. Zhong, Zheng, Li et al., "Epidemiology and Cause of Severe Acute Respiratory Syndrome (SARS) in Guangdong, People's Republic of China, in February, 2003." See also N. Lee, D. Hui, A. Wu et al., "A Major Outbreak of Severe Acute Respiratory Syndrome in Hong Kong." *New England Journal of Medicine,* 348 (2003): 1986–94.

41. R. P. Wenzel and M. B. Edmond, "Managing SARS Amidst Uncertainty," *New England Journal of Medicine* 348 (2003): 1947–48.

42. C. Abraham, "Fateful Encounter Tied to Spread of Mystery Bug; Officials Think Victims Caught Pneumonia While Waiting for Elevator in Hong Kong," *Globe and Mail,* March 21, 2003.

43. M. Pottinger, "Hong Kong Hotel Was a Virus Hub—Doctor from China Passed Germ to Others, Who Then Moved on to Other Nations," *Wall Street Journal,* March 21, 2003, B2.

44. Abraham, "Fateful Encounter."

45. P. Orwen and G. Swainson, "Deadly Illness in York: Officials," *Toronto Star,* March 17, 2003.

46. K. Faught, "Quick Response to Contain a Killer—Isolation of Second Toronto Victim Credited. Scientists Say They May Have Test for Mysterious Illness," *Toronto Star,* March 22, 2003.

47. C. Abraham, "Mystery Bug May Spread More Easily Than Expected; Canadian Patient Contracts SARS Disease After Sharing Hospital Room with Victim," *Globe and Mail,* March 19, 2003.

48. T. Svobada, B. Henry, L. Shulman et al., "Public Health Measures to Control the Spread of the Severe Acute Respiratory Syndrome During the Outbreak in Toronto," *New England Journal of Medicine* 350 (2004): 2352–61.

49. Abraham, "Mystery Bug."

50. C. Abraham, "Canadian Laboratory Zeros in on SARS Virus; Winnipeg Scientists Find Same Pathogen in Samples from Six Patients with Disease," *Globe and Mail,* March 22, 2003.

51. C. Abraham, "Mystery Ailment Feared in 14 Health Workers," *Globe and Mail,* March 25, 2003.

52. A. Picard, "Scientists Seek to Solve Puzzle of SARS Pathogen," *Globe and Mail,* March 28, 2003.

53. T. Kalinowski. "SARS Claims Third Toronto Life—Illness Kills Man Who Shared Room With Earlier Victim. Two New Cases of Acute Pneumonia Are Suspected." *Toronto Star,* March 23, 2003.

54. J. Mawhinney and P. Mascoll, "Mystery Bug Shuts Hospital Emergency Room," *Toronto Star,* March 24, 2003.

55. C. Abraham, "Premier Declares Health Emergency; The SARS Alert: Every Person Who's Been to One Toronto Hospital Since March 16 Is Told to Stay

Inside, as Officials Scramble to Contain a Puzzling Infectious Ailment," *Globe and Mail,* March 27, 2003.

56. T. Perkins, "SARS Fears Shut Down Toronto School; Parents Alerted After Three Pupils in Kindergarten Hit by High Fevers," *Globe and Mail,* March 26, 2003.

57. K. Palmer and T. Talaga, "Bug Fuels Quarantine Alert—25 Families Confined but Dozens May Follow; MD Says School Closed and Travelers Told to Delay Asian Trips," *Toronto Star,* March 26, 2003.

58. A. Picard and C. Alphonso, "Canada Pressed to Screen Travelers; Health Body Worried by SARS Outbreak; Toronto Hospitals Closed to Most Visitors," *Globe and Mail,* March 28, 2003.

59. J. Wong, "Screened for SARS at Pearson Blasted; Doctor, Nurse Returning from China Trip Say Official Precautions Were Totally Inadequate," *Globe and Mail,* March 29, 2003.

60. C. Alphonso, "Ottawa Tries to Erase Toronto's Black Eye; The SARS Outbreak: Anger and Appeals Greet a Surprise Advisory Telling the World to Avoid the City," *Globe and Mail,* April 24, 2003. See also J. Lewington and J. Rusk, "Mayor Calls Advisory Devastating; Tourism Officials Join City Leader in Plan to Reduce Economic Fallout of WHO Edict," *Globe and Mail,* April 24, 2003.

61. Interview on www.cnn.com, "SARS According to Mayor Mel," *Globe and Mail,* April 26, 2003.

62. E. Oziewicz, "Why the WHO Took Action; Two Deaths in Philippines Show How One Case Can Spread SARS, Official Says," *Globe and Mail,* April 25, 2003.

63. Ibid.

64. A. Picard and C. Alphonso, "Canadians Ratchet Up Criticism of Travel Advisory," *Globe and Mail,* April 25, 2003.

65. J. Lewington, "Blitz Aims to Calm Fears of SARS, Get Tourists Back," *Globe and Mail,* April 25, 2003.

66. N. Keung, K. Palmer, and B. Powell, "City Seeks Clean Bill of Health— SARS Economic Toll Wearies Business, Workers Ad Campaign Hopes to Bring out Big Spenders," *Toronto Star,* May 10, 2003.

67. The travel advisory lasted six days.

68. G. MacDonald and O. Moore, "Shadow of SARS Is Lifted; As Canada Is Taken off the WHO's List, Plans to Rebuild Toronto's Shattered Image Centre on Tourism, and the Rolling Stones," *Globe and Mail,* May 15, 2003.

69. O. Moore, "Toronto Hit with SARS Bombshell; Four More People Believed Stricken; Hundreds Asked to Go into Quarantine," *Globe and Mail,* May 23, 2003.

70. C. Abraham and L. Priest, "SARS: How The Quest for a Quick Victory Led to Costly Error," *Globe and Mail,* May 31, 2003.

71. C. Alphonso, "SARS-Stricken Toronto Likely Back on WHO List," *Globe and Mail,* May 26, 2003.

72. G. Galloway, "Scope of SARS Outbreak Understated, Critics Say; Two More Patients Die as Controversy Grows over Actions of Health," *Globe and Mail,* May 29, 2003.

73. Svobada, Shulman et al., "Public Health Measures."

74. Galloway, "Scope of SARS Outbreak Understated, Critics Say."

75. T. Boyle, "SARS-Weary Nurses Demand Danger Pay—Private Hires Blamed for Morale Drop; Agency Nurses Get $100/Hr., Others $21," *The Toronto Star,* May 29, 2003. See also T. Talaga, "Government 'Dropped The Ball,' Nurse Charges—No Relief in Sight for Weary Workers. Restrictions Eased Too Soon: Nurse," *The Toronto Star,* May 28, 2003.

76. Talaga, "Government 'Dropped The Ball'."

77. Ibid.

78. The SARS Commission. http://www.sarscommission.ca/index.html.

79. M. Wente, "A Lame-Duck Embarrassment? No-o-o-body but Mel," *Globe and Mail,* May 8, 2003.

80. Editorial, "Where Are the Leaders When They're Needed?" *Globe and Mail,* April 25, 2003.

81. City of Toronto, City Councillors. http://www.toronto.ca/councillors/ootes1.htm.

82. Chief Administrator's Office, Strategic & Corporate Policy Division, "Amalgamation in the City of Toronto. A Case Study," Montreal, Canada, April 8, 2004. ejc.inrs-ucs.uquebec.ca/Toronto.pdf.

83. Case Ootes, Councillor in charge of Ward 29, Toronto-Danforth, telephone interview, March 16, 2007.

84. Kahn and Barondess, "Preparing for Disaster."

CHAPTER 5: SUCCESS FAVORS THE PREPARED PUBLIC HEALTH LEADER

1. Institute of Medicine, *The Future of Public Health* (Washington, DC: National Academy Press, 1988), 102–4.

2. Dr. Daksh Patel (physician in private practice), telephone interview, June 28, 2007.

3. Christy Stephenson (former president and CEO of Robert Wood Johnson University Hospital at Hamilton), telephone interview, March 28, 2007. Stephenson began her career as a registered nurse.

4. Governor Christine Todd Whitman left New Jersey to become the head of the U.S. Environmental Protection Agency on January 31, 2001. Acting Governor Donald DiFrancesco took over until James McGreevey was sworn into office on January 15, 2002.

5. Anthrax, a bacterium that can turn itself into hardy spores, can infect a body either through a breach in the skin (cutaneous anthrax), through contaminated food (gastrointestinal anthrax), or through inhalation into the lungs (inhalational anthrax—the most deadly type of anthrax infection).

6. Dr. George T. DiFerdinando, Jr. (former acting commissioner of New Jersey Department of Health and Senior Services), telephone interview, June 11, 2007.

7. T.V. Inglesby, D.A. Henderson, J.G. Bartlett et al., "Anthrax as a Biological Weapon," *JAMA* 281 (1999): 1735–45.

8. Dr. Larry Bush (infectious disease specialist in private practice in Florida), telephone interview, June 11, 2007.

9. Dr. Jean Marie Malecki (director, Palm Beach County Health Department, Florida), telephone interview January 26, 2007.

10. Dr. Georges Benjamin (executive director, American Public Health Association), telephone interview, June 28, 2007.

11. Dr. Margaret Hamburg was the New York City commissioner of health from 1991 to 1997.

12. Dr. Steve Ostroff was the associate director for epidemiological science, National Center for Infectious Diseases, CDC.

13. Dr. Neal L. Cohen (New York City commissioner of health and mental hygiene during the anthrax crisis), telephone interview, August 9, 2007.

14. West Allis is a suburb of Milwaukee, WI. http://www.ci.west-allis.wi.us/.

15. Dr. Thomas Taft (infectious disease specialist in private practice in Milwaukee, Wisconsin), telephone interview, June 14, 2007.

16. Paul Nannis (commissioner of health of Milwaukee during 1993 *cryptosporidium* outbreak), telephone interview, January 16, 2007. Nannis graduated from the University of Wisconsin, Milwaukee, with a master's degree in social work. The University of Wisconsin honored him with a distinguished alumni award. http://www.uwm.edu/News/PR/05.05/UWMAAawards.html.

17. ProMED is an online global infectious disease and toxin surveillance system run by the International Society for Infectious Diseases. http://www.promed mail.org/pls/promed/f?p=2400:1000:12583842145158663484.

18. Dr. Donald Low (microbiologist-in-chief, Department of Microbiology, Mount Sinai Hospital, Toronto), telephone interview, May 29, 2007.

19. Dr. Bonnie Henry (associate medical officer of health in Toronto during 2003 SARS crisis), telephone interview, April 19, 2007. (Dr. Sheela Basrur was appointed chief medical officer of health for the province of Ontario. After the outbreak, she had to resign her position after developing a rare form of cancer. http://www.canada.com/topics/news/national/story.html?id=4be69cf9-19ae-42cd-b0e2-5d3206119af1&k=73430.

20. J.D. Aberbach, R.D. Putnam, and B.A. Rockman, *Bureaucrats and Politicians in Western Democracies* (Cambridge, MA: Harvard University Press, 1981), 1–23.

21. Ibid.

CHAPTER 6: CONFRONTING UNCERTAINTY

1. J.C. Gaydos, F.H. Top, Jr., R.A. Hodder et al., "Swine Influenza A Outbreak, Fort Dix, New Jersey, 1976," *Emerging Infectious Diseases* 12 (2006): 23–28. The novel virus was classified as A/New Jersey/76 (Hsw1N1, which is now classified as H1N1).

2. Ibid. See also R.E. Neustadt, and H. Fineberg, *The Epidemic That Never Was—Policy-Making & the Swine Flue Affair* (New York and Toronto: Random House, 1982): 18–19. The 1918 virus has recently been reconstructed and has been

shown to be of avian, not swine, origin (T. M. Tumpey, C. F. Basler, P. V. Aguilar et al., "Characterization of the Reconstructed 1918 Spanish Influenza Pandemic Virus," *Science* 310 (2005): 77–80). It is now understood that wild waterfowl, such as geese and ducks, are the natural hosts of the influenza A virus and the source for human pandemics. Influenza A viruses have two different proteins on their surface: hemagglutinin (H) and neuraminidase (N). There are 16 different H proteins (numbered 1 to 16), and 9 different N proteins (numbered 1 to 9). The viruses change by mixing different H and N proteins such as H1N1 and H5N1. http://www.cdc.gov/flu/about/viruses/types.htm.

See M. C. Zambon, "Epidemiology and Pathogenesis of Influenza," *Journal of Antimicrobial Chemotherapy* 44 (1999): 3–9.

3. E. D. Kilbourne, "Flu to the Starboard! Man the Harpoons! Fill 'em with Vaccine! Get the Captain! Hurry!" *New York Times,* February 13, 1976, 32.

4. H. M. Schmeck Jr., "U.S. Calls Flu Alert on Possible Return of Epidemic's Virus," *New York Times,* February 20, 1976, 1.

5. Ibid.

6. Neustadt, and Fineberg, *The Epidemic That Never Was,* 17–31.

7. Ibid.

8. D. J. Sencer and J. D. Millar, "Reflections on the 1976 Swine Flu Vaccination Program," *Emerging Infectious Diseases* 12 (2006): 29–33.

9. Ibid.

10. Ibid.

11. Gaydos, Top, Hodder, et al., "Swine Influenza,"

12. Sencer and Millar, "Reflections."

13. Neustadt and Fineberg, *The Epidemic That Never Was,* 173, 187.

14. Sencer and Millar, "Reflections." See also A. D. Langmuir, D. J. Bregman, L. T. Kurland et al., "An Epidemiologic and Clinical Evaluation of Guillain-Barré Syndrome Reported in Association with the Administration of Swine Influenza Vaccines," *American Journal of Epidemiology* 119 (1984): 841–79.

15. Langmuir, Bregman, and Kurland, "An Epidemiologic and Clinical Evaluation." Guillain-Barré syndrome is a rare disorder in which the body's immune system attacks the peripheral nerves and can cause paralysis and death. The disease is a medical emergency and can require weeks in intensive care until movement is regained. The cause is unknown although viral respiratory and gastrointestinal infections as well as vaccinations and surgery have preceded onset.

16. A. B. Sabin, "Washington and the Flu," *New York Times,* November 5, 1976, 21. (Typical influenza seasons run from September or October to March.)

17. Ibid.

18. H. Schwartz, "Swine Flu Fiasco," *New York Times,* December 21, 1976, 33.

19. Neustadt and Fineberg, *The Epidemic that Never Was,* 5.

20. R. Krause, "The Swine Flu Episode and the Fog of Epidemics," *Emerging Infectious Diseases* 12 (2006): 40–43.

21. Sencer and Millar, "Reflections."

22. David J. Sencer (former director of CDC during swine flu outbreak, 1976–77), telephone interview, November 6, 2006.

23. There are two major types of influenza: type A and type B. Only type A is capable of causing pandemics, (http://www.cdc.gov/flu/about/viruses/index.htm). Because wild waterfowl, such as ducks, are the natural hosts of influenza A viruses, they can never be eradicated.

24. K. S. Li, Y, Guan, J. Wang et al., "Genesis of a Highly Pathogenic and Potentially Pandemic H5N1 Influenza Virus in Eastern Asia," *Nature* 430 (2004): 209–13.

25. J. S. Tam, "Influenza A (H5N1) in Hong Kong: An Overview," *Vaccine* 20 (2002): S77–S81.

26. *Deutsche Presse-Agentur,* "Experts Hold Urgent Meetings as "Bird Flu" Continues to Kill People," December 7, 1997.

27. *Deutsche Presse-Agentur,* "Hong Kong Health Department Issues Guidelines amid bird flu scare," December 8, 1997.

28. E. A. Gargan, "Chicken-Borne Flu Virus Puts Hong Kong on Alert," *New York Times,* December 17, 1997, A6.

29. S. Buerk and B. Wong Wai-Yuk, "Border Alert on Poultry; Anson Chan Announces Taskforce to Keep Public Informed About Virus," *South China Morning Post* (Hong Kong), December 14, 1997, 1.

30. *South China Morning Post,* "Farmers May Kill Million Chickens," December 21, 1997, 3.

31. Editorial, "Clear Message Needed," *South China Morning Post* (Hong Kong), December 21, 1997.

32. Associated Press, "Mass Slaughter of Chickens Set; Hong Kong Orders 1.2 Million Birds Killed to Battle Flu," *Toronto Star,* December 29, 1997, A1. See also Reuters News Agency, "Million Chickens Face Axe to Halt Flu; Hong Kong Bans Birds from China," *Globe and Mail* (Canada), December 29, 1997, A1.

33. S. Lee, "Slaughter Held Up by Inexperience," *South China Morning Post* (Hong Kong), December 31, 1997, 3.

34. *South China Morning Post* (Hong Kong), "Killings: Errors Admitted," January 3, 1998, 1. See also K. B. Richburg, "Chicken Sightings Frighten Hong Kong; Criticism Rises as Officials Admit Mishandling of 'Bird Flu' Crisis," *South China Morning Post* (Hong Kong), January 3, 1998, A1.

35. Editorial, "Taking Charge," *South China Morning Post* (Hong Kong), January 3, 1998, 14.

36. M. Shuchman, "Improving Global Health—Margaret Chan at the WHO," *New England Journal of Medicine* 356 (2007): 653–56. See also K. S. Li, Y. Guan, J. Wang et al., "Genesis of a Highly Pathogenic and Potentially Pandemic H5N1 Influenza Virus in Eastern Asia," *Nature* 430 (2004): 209–13.

37. Writing Committee of the World Health Organization (WHO) Consultation on Human Influenza A/H5, "Avian Influenza A (H5N1) Infection in Humans," *New England Journal of Medicine* 353 (2005): 1374–85.

38. Writing Committee of the Second World Health Organization Consultation on Clinical Aspects of Human Infection with Avian Influenza A (H5N1) Virus, "Update on Avian Influenza A (H5N1) Virus Infection in Humans," *New England Journal of Medicine,* 2008; 358 (2008): 261–73.

39. World Health Organization, "Cumulative Number of Confirmed Human Cases of Avian Influenza A (H5N1) Reported to WHO," June 1, 2009. http://www.who.int/csr/disease/avian_influenza/country/cases_table_2009_06_01/en/index.html.

40. Writing Committee of the Second World Health Organization, "Update on Avian Influenza A (H5N1) Virus Infection in Humans. *New England Journal of Medicine* 358 (2008): 261–73.

41. World Health Organization World Health Organization, "Cumulative Number of Confirmed Human Cases of Avian Influenza A (H5N1) Reported to WHO," June 2, 2009. http://www.who.int/csr/disease/avian_influenza/country/cases_table_2009_06_02/en/index.html

42. A. Sipress, "Indonesia Neglected Bird Flu Until Too Late, Experts Say," *Washington Post,* October 20, 2005, A1.

43. Ibid.

44. A. Sipress, "Urging Indonesia to Take Stronger Action Against Bird Flu," *Washington Post,* October 23, 2005, A19.

45. Alan Sipress (journalist, *Washington Post*), telephone interview, January 31, 2008.

46. Centers for Disease Control, "Outbreak of Swine-Origin Influenza A (H1N1) Virus Infection—Mexico, March-April 2009," *Morbidity and Mortality Weekly Report* 58 (May 8, 2009): 467–70. http://www.cdc.gov/mmwr/preview/mmwr html/mm5817a5.htm.

47. J. Partlow and W. Booth, "Poverty, Tendency to Self-Medicate Help Drive up Flu Deaths in Mexico," *Washington Post*, May 5, 2009. http://www.washing tonpost.com/wp-dyn/content/article/2009/05/04/AR2009050403755.html.

48. After China initially denied and then downplayed the 2003 SARS crisis, the global public health community realized that the international health regulations (IHR), which had been last updated in 1969, had to be revised. The World Health Assembly approved new regulations on May 23, 2005 that entered into force July 18, 2007. The new international agreement was designed to contain or prevent serious risks to public health and discourage unnecessary restrictions on trade or travel. WHO member states must notify WHO within 48 hours of any threat that qualifies as a public health emergency of international concern. The 2009 swine flu epidemic is the first international disease crisis to occur under the new IHR. http://www.who.int/ihr/en/.

49. Novel Swine-Origin Influenza A (H1N1) Virus Investigation Team. "Emergence of a Novel Swine-Origin Influenza A (H1N1) Virus in Humans," *New England Journal of Medicine* 361 (2009). http://content.nejm.org/cgi/content/full/NEJ Moa0903810v1.

50. M. Lacey and E. Malkin. "Mexico Takes Powers to Isolate Cases of Swine Flu," *New York Times* April 26, 2009. http://www.nytimes.com/2009/04/26/world/americas/26mexico.html.

51. Pandemic phase four occurs when there are small clusters of disease with limited human-to-human spread. WHO categorized the ongoing avian influenza crisis at pandemic phase four. Phase five occurs when human-to-human spread is

still localized, but the clusters of disease are larger. Phase six is a pandemic with increased and sustained disease transmission in the general population. http://www. who.int/csr/disease/influenza/GIPA3AideMemoire.pdf.

52. L. H. Kahn, "Who's in Charge During the Swine Flu Crisis?" *Bulletin of the Atomic Scientists* (April 29, 2009). http://www.thebulletin.org/web-edition/col umnists/laura-h-kahn/whos-charge-during-the-swine-flu-crisis.

53. S. Murray, "Sebelius Confirmed as Secretary of HHS," *Washington Post*, April 28, 2009. http://voices.washingtonpost.com/44/2009/04/28/sebelius_confir mation_expected.html.

54. A. Browne, "China Forces Dozens of Mexican Travelers into Quarantine," *Wall Street Journal*, May 4, 2009. http://online.wsj.com/article/SB124137876 507580987.html.

55. N. Audi, "Culling Pigs in Flu Fight, Egypt Angers Herders and Dismays U.N.," *New York Times*, May 1, 2009. http://www.nytimes.com/2009/05/01/ health/01egypt.html.

56. S. S. Hsu, "U.S. Warns Other Nations Not to Ban Pork," *Washington Post*, April 29, 2009. http://www.washingtonpost.com/wp-dyn/content/article/2009/04/ 28/AR2009042801442.html.

57. World Animal Health Organization, "The OIE Strongly Counsels Against the Culling of Pigs," *Press Release*, April 30, 2009. http://www.oie.int/eng/ press/en_090430.htm.

58. *Washington Post*, "Foot-in-Mouth Disease," May 1, 2009. http://www.wash ingtonpost.com/wp-dyn/content/article/2009/04/30/AR2009043002660.html.

59. E. Malkin and S. Otterman, "Mexico Prepares to Lower Alert as Flu Cases Ebb," *New York Times*. May 5, 2009. http://www.nytimes.com/2009/05/05/health/ 05flu.html?_r=1&partner=rss&emc=rss.

60. A. E. Cha, "Caught in China's Aggressive Swine Flu Net. Quarantine Mea sures Keep Cases Down but Virtually Imprison Healthy Travelers," *Washington Post*, May 29, 2009. http://www.washingtonpost.com/wp-dyn/content/article/ 2009/05/28/AR2009052803919_pf.html.

61. D. G. McNeil Jr., "W.H.O. Raises Alert Level as Flu Spreads to 74 Countries," *New York Times*, June 12, 2009. http://www.nytimes.com/2009/06/12/world/ asia/12flu.html?hp.

62. World Health Organization, "Influenza A (H1N1)—update 47." June 11, 2009. http://www.who.int/csr/don/2009_06_11/en/index.html.

63. T. T. Wang and P. Palese, "Unraveling the Mystery of Swine Influenza Virus," *Cell* June 12, 2009; 137: 983–985.

64. P. Palese, "Why Swine Flu Isn't So Scary," *Wall Street Journal*, May 2, 2009. http://online.wsj.com/article/SB124122223484879119.html.

65. T. T. Wang and P. Palese, "Unraveling the Mystery of Swine Influenza Vi rus," *Cell* 137 (June 12, 2009): 983–85.

66. L. T. White, "SARS, Anti-Populism, and Elite Lies: Diseases from Which China Can Recover," in *The New Global Threat: Severe Acute Respiratory Dis tress Syndrome and Its Impacts,* ed. T. Koh (Singapore: World Scientific Press, 2003), 31–68.

67. World Health Organization. SARS. http://www.wpro.who.int/health_top ics/sars/.

68. G. Bates, "Contagious Confusion: China Will Pay Dearly for SARS Debacle," *International Herald Tribune,* April 22, 2003. http://www.iht.com/articles/2003/04/22/edgill_ed3_.php.

69. M. Enserink, "Riding the Biodefense Wave," *Science* 301 (2003): 912–13.

70. KPCB News, "Thomas Monath, M.D. to Join Kleiner Perkins Caufield & Byers to Advance Innovation in Infectious Diseases with the New KPCB Pandemic and Bio Defense Fund." http://www.kpcb.com/news/articles/2006_05_17.html.

71. "Arbovirus" is an abbreviation for arthropod-borne virus, which is a virus transmitted by insects such as mosquitoes.

72. Dr. Thomas Monath, personal e-mail communication, July 17, 2007.

73. Dr. Lawrence Kerr, personal e-mail communication, February 17, 2008.

74. There were two French scandals involving HIV-tainted blood. First, in the early 1980s, thousands of people were given HIV-tainted blood because French government officials delayed approving a U.S. screening test in order to let a domestic French company develop a similar product. Screening of blood was not obligatory until August 1985. The second scandal emerged in 1991 when three former health officials were convicted of fraud and criminal negligence for delaying the introduction of heat treatment for blood products. They allowed approximately 1,500 hemophiliacs to become infected with HIV from contaminated clotting factor. Institut Merieux, a French drug company, subsequently acknowledged that as late as November 1985, it exported unsterilized and untested blood products after knowing about the dangers. Then French Prime Minister Pierre Beregovoy moved to back a constitutional amendment that would make it easier to bring cabinet officials to justice for offenses committed while in office. In 1999, former French Prime Minister Laurent Fabius and his ex-minister of social affairs Georgina Dufoix were acquitted of manslaughter, but the former health minister, Edmond Herve, was convicted. Fabius argued that as prime minister, he could not have had the expertise to decide on such a complicated issue as the new AIDS disease. *New York Times,* "French Cabinet Imposes Curbs After Blood Scandal," November 2, 1992. http://query.nytimes.com/gst/fullpage.html?res=9E0CE7D81 531F936A35752C1A964958260. See also *BBC News,* "Europe: Blood Scandal Ministers Walk Free," March 9, 1999. http://news.bbc.co.uk/2/hi/europe/293367. stm; and T. Patel, "France Faces Fresh HIV Blood Scandal, *New Scientist,* February 1994. http://www.newscientist.com/article/mg14119130.800-france-faces-fresh-hiv-blood-scandal-.html.

75. Dr. Jean-Claude Manuguerra, personal interview, March 11, 2008.

76. Professor Lord Robert May, telephone interview, May 27, 2008.

77. P.A. Rota, M.S. Oberste, S.S. Monroe et al., "Characterization of a Novel Coronavirus Associated with Severe Acute Respiratory Syndrome," *Science* 300 (2003): 1394–99.

78. R.M. Anderson, C. Fraser, A.C. Ghani et al., "Epidemiology, Transmission Dynamics and Control of SARS: The 2002–2003 Epidemic," *Philosophical Transactions of the Royal Society B: Biological Sciences,* 359 (2004): 1091–1105. http://journals.royalsociety.org/content/x548y4tcmyweu7ra/fulltext.pdf.

79. W. Li, Z. Shi, and M. Yu, "Bats Are Natural Reservoirs of SARS-Like Coronaviruses," *Science,* 310 (2005): 676–79.

80. M. Enserink, "Reports Blame Animal Health Lab in Foot-and-Mouth Whodunit," *Science,* 317 (2007): 1486.

81. "Incubation period" is the time interval between exposure and the development of symptoms.

82. WHO Writing Group, "Nonpharmaceutical Interventions for Pandemic Influenza, National and Community Measures," *Emerging Infectious Diseases* 12 (2006): 88–94. http://www.cdc.gov/ncidod/eid/vol12no01/05-1371.htm.

83. L. Garrett and D. P. Fidler, "Sharing H5N1 Viruses to Stop a Global Influenza Pandemic," *PloS Medicine* 4 (2007): 1712–14. http://medicine.plosjournals.org/perlserv/?request=get-document&doi=10.1371%2Fjournal.pmed.0040330.

84. J. Knight, "Clear as Mud," *Nature* 423 (2003): 376–78.

CHAPTER 7: THE VITAL LINK BETWEEN ANIMAL AND HUMAN HEALTH, PART I

1. M. Palmarini, "A Veterinary Twist on Pathogen Biology," *PloS Pathogens* 3 (2007): e12. http://dx.doi.org/10.1371/journal.ppat.0030012.

2. M. E. J. Woolhouse, P. Coen, L. Matthews et al., "A Centuries-Long Epidemic of Scrapie in British Sheep?" *Trends in Microbiology* 9 (2001): 67–70. The disease was called "scrapie" because the affected animals would scrape themselves against fences, trees, and other hard surfaces in attempts to relieve itching.

3. T. Alper, W. A. Cramp, D. A. Haig, and M. C. Clarke, "Does the Agent of Scrapie Replicate Without Nucleic Acid?" *Nature,* 214 (1967): 764–66.

4. S. B. Prusiner, "Novel Proteinaceous Infectious Particles Cause Scrapie," *Science,* 216 (1982): 136–44.

5. M. Jeffrey, I. A. Goodbrand, and C. M. Goodsir, "Pathology of the Transmissible Spongiform Encephalopathies with Special Emphasis on Ultrastructures," *Micron,* 26 (1995): 277–98.

6. *The BSE Inquiry: The Inquiry into BSE and Variant CJD in the United Kingdom.* Vol. 2. Science. 2. The Spongiform Encephalopathies—knowledge existing in 1986. Transmission of TSEs. http://www.bseinquiry.gov.uk/report/volume2/chapteri.htm#818094.

7. *The BSE Inquiry.* Vol. 3: The Early Years, 1986–88. Section 1. The identification of a new disease in cattle. The earliest confirmed case. http://www.bseinquiry.gov.uk/report/volume3/chapterd.htm.

8. Ibid.

9. A nyala is a South African antelope that belongs to the family Bovidae. The Bovidae family includes wild animals such as antelopes, bison, buffalo, as well as domesticated animals such as cattle, goats, and sheep.

10. M. Jeffrey and G. Wells, "Spongiform Encephalopathy in a Nyala (Tragelaphus angasi)," *Veterinary Pathology* 25 (1988): 398–99.

11. *The BSE Inquiry.* Vol. 3: The Early Years, 1986–88. Section 2. Dissemination of information. June 1986. http://www.bseinquiry.gov.uk/report/volume3/chaptea4.htm.

12. *The BSE Inquiry.* Vol. 3: The Early Years, 1986–88. Section 1. The identification of a new disease in cattle. The identification of the emergence of BSE. http://www.bseinquiry.gov.uk/report/volume3/chapterf.htm#515721.

13. Ibid.

14. *The BSE Inquiry.* Vol. 2: Science. Section 3. The nature and cause of BSE. The investigation of the BSE epidemic. http://www.bseinquiry.gov.uk/report/volume2/chapteb2.htm.

15. *The BSE Inquiry.* Vol. 3: The Early Years, 1986–88. Section 2. Dissemination of information. June 1987. http://www.bseinquiry.gov.uk/report/volume3/chaptea5.htm.

16. Ibid.

17. G. A. Wells, A. C. Scott, C. T. Johnson et al. "A Novel Progressive Spongiform Encephalopathy in Cattle," *Veterinary Record* 121 (1987): 419–20.

18. *The BSE Inquiry.* Vol. 3: The Early Years, 1986–88. http://www.bseinquiry.gov.uk/report/volume3/chapterd.htm#512980.

19. *The BSE Inquiry.* Vol. 16: Reference Material. BSE chronology. http://www.bseinquiry.gov.uk/report/volume16/chapter1.htm.

20. *The BSE Inquiry.* Vol. 1: Findings and Conclusions. 4. The Southwood Working Party and other scientific advisory committees. http://www.bseinquiry.gov.uk/report/volume1/chapter4.htm.

21. P. Aldhous, "Inquiry Blames Missed Warnings for Scale of Britain's BSE Crisis," *Nature,* 408 (2000): 3–5.

22. *The BSE Inquiry.* Vol. 3: The Early Years, 1986–88. 3. Epidemiology. The feed industry consulted. http://www.bseinquiry.gov.uk/report/volume3/chapteb5.htm#547293.

23. *The BSE Inquiry.* Vol. 4: The Southwood Working Party, 1988–89. 4. Preparations for the second meeting. http://www.bseinquiry.gov.uk/report/volume4/chapter4.htm.

24. *The BSE Inquiry.* Vol. 1: Findings and Conclusions. 4. The Southwood Working Party and other scientific advisory committees. http://www.bseinquiry.gov.uk/report/volume1/chapter4.htm.

25. *The BSE Inquiry.* Vol. 3: The Early Years, 1986–88. 4. The ruminant feed ban. Mr. MacGregor's decision. http://www.bseinquiry.gov.uk/report/volume3/chaptec2.htm.

26. *The BSE Inquiry.* Vol. 3: The Early Years, 1986–88. 4. The ruminant feed ban. The meeting with the industry. http://www.bseinquiry.gov.uk/report/volume3/chaptec3.htm.

27. *The BSE Inquiry.* Vol. 3: The Early Years, 1986–88. 4. The ruminant feed ban. The decision to grant a period of grace. http://www.bseinquiry.gov.uk/report/volume3/chaptec4.htm.

28. *The BSE Inquiry.* Vol. 4: The Southwood Working Party, 1988–89. 4. Preparations for the second meeting. http://www.bseinquiry.gov.uk/report/volume4/chapter4.htm.

29. Ibid. See also *The BSE Inquiry.* Vol. 2: Science. 3. The nature and cause of BSE. http://www.bseinquiry.gov.uk/report/volume2/chapteb2.htm#820216; and

H. Fraser, M. E. Bruce, A. Chree et al., " Transmission of Bovine Spongiform Encephalopathy and Scrapie to Mice," *Journal of General Virology* 73 (1992): 1891–97.

30. J. W. Wilesmith, G. A. H. Wells, M. P. Cranwell, and J. B. M. Ryan, "Bovine Spongiform Encephalopathy: Epidemiological Studies," *The Veterinary Record* 123 (1988): 638–44. See also *The BSE Inquiry.* Vol. 3: The Early Years, 1986–88. 3. Epidemiology. The feed industry consulted. http://www.bseinquiry.gov.uk/report/volume3/chapteb5.htm#547293.

31. *The BSE Inquiry.* Vol. 3: The Early Years, 1986–88. 3. Epidemiology. Changes in the production processes of MBM identified. http://www.bseinquiry.gov.uk/report/volume3/chapteb6.htm. See also Wilesmith et al., "Bovine Spongiform Encephalopathy." The rendering process involves drying and cooking the discarded parts of animal carcasses, including organs and entrails, to make MBM and tallow.

32. Wilesmith et al., "Bovine Spongiform Encephalopathy."

33. William Hueston (professor at the School of Public Health and College of Veterinary Medicine, University of Minnesota; member of SEAC 1993–99), personal email communication, February 12, 2009.

34. J. W. Wilesmith, "An Epidemiologist's View of Bovine Spongiform Encephalopathy," *Philosophical Transaction of the Royal Society of London B* 343 (1994): 357–61.

35. *The BSE Inquiry.* Vol. 4: The Southwood Working Party, 1988–89. 4. Preparations for the second meeting. http://www.bseinquiry.gov.uk/report/volume4/chapter4.htm.

36. *The BSE Inquiry.* Vol. 16: Reference Material. BSE chronology. http://www.bseinquiry.gov.uk/report/volume16/chapter1.htm.

37. *The BSE Inquiry.* Vol. 1: Findings and Conclusions. 4. The Southwood Working Party and other scientific advisory committees. The Southwood Working Party. http://www.bseinquiry.gov.uk/report/volume1/chapter4.htm#643916.

38. Ibid.

39. *The BSE Inquiry.* Vol. 8: Variant CJD. 5. Emergence of variant CJD. Discussion on the work of the CJD Surveillance Unit (CJDSU). http://www.bseinquiry.gov.uk/report/volume8/chapteb6.htm.

40. *The BSE Inquiry.* Vol. 6: Human Health, 1989–96. 3. Introduction of the ban on specified bovine offal. Overview of events in 1989. http://www.bseinquiry.gov.uk/report/volume6/chapte32.htm.

41. The committee included Dr. David Tyrrell, chair; Professor John Bourne, director of the Institute for Animal Health; Dr. Richard Kimberlin, former director of the NPU in Edinburgh and head of the Scrapie and Related Diseases Advisory Service; Dr. William Watson, director of the CVL, MAFF; and Dr. Robert Will, a consultant neurologist at the Western General Hospital, Edinburgh. http://www.bseinquiry.gov.uk/report/volume11/chapter2.htm#45919.

42. *The BSE Inquiry.* Vol. 11: Scientists after Southwood. 3. The Tyrrell Report. Development of the report. http://www.bseinquiry.gov.uk/report/volume11/chapteb2.htm.

43. The UK Medical Research Council is a publicly funded organization that supports research to improve human health. http://www.mrc.ac.uk/index.htm.

44. *The BSE Inquiry.* Vol. 11: Scientists after Southwood. 3. The Tyrrell Report. Final publication. http://www.bseinquiry.gov.uk/report/volume11/chaptea6.htm#51891.

45. *The BSE Inquiry.* Vol. 11: Scientists after Southwood. 4. The Spongiform Encephalopathy Advisory Committee (SEAC). Establishment of SEAC. http://www.bseinquiry.gov.uk/report/volume11/chapter4.htm.

46. *The BSE Inquiry.* Vol. 8: Variant CJD. 3. Establishment of the CJD Surveillance Unit. http://www.bseinquiry.gov.uk/report/volume8/chapteb2.htm.

47. Will Hueston, personal email communication, February 12, 2009.

48. Ibid.

49. R. G. Will, J. W. Ironside, M. Zeidler et al., "A New Variant of Creutzfeldt-Jakob Disease in the U.K.," *The Lancet* 347 (1996): 921–25. See also J. Almond and J. Pattison, "Human BSE," *Nature* 389 (1997): 437–38; and *The BSE Inquiry.* Vol. 16: Reference Material. BSE chronology. http://www.bseinquiry.gov.uk/report/volume16/chron2.htm.

50. E. Beghi, C. Gandolfo, C. Ferrarese et al., "Bovine Spongiform Encephalopathy and Creutzfeldt-Jakob Disease: Facts and Uncertainties Underlying the Causal Link Between Animal and Human Diseases," *Neurological Science* 25 (2004): 122–29.

51. Ibid.

52. A. F. Hill, M. Desbruslais, S. Joiner et al., "The Same Prion Strain Causes vCJD and BSE," *Nature,* 389 (1997): 448–50. See also M. E. Bruce, R. G. Will, J. W. Ironside, et al., "Transmissions to Mice Indicate That 'New Variant' CJD Is Caused by the BSE Agent," *Nature* 389 (1997): 498–501.

53. Editorial, "Less Beef, More Brain," *The Lancet* 347 (1996): 915.

54. *The BSE Inquiry.* Home. http://www.bseinquiry.gov.uk/index.htm.

55. P. Aldhous, "Inquiry Blames Missed Warnings for Scale of Britain's BSE Crisis," *Nature* 408 (2000): 3–5.

56. H. Ashraf, "The Phillips Report on BSE and vCJD," *The Lancet* 356 (2000): 1579–80.

57. P. Van Zwanenberg and E. Millstone, *BSE: Risk, Science, and Governance* (Oxford, UK: Oxford University Press, 2005).

58. Sir John Pattison, dean of University College London Medical School and Professor of Medical Microbiology. SEAC chair since November 1995. House of Lords—Select Committee on Science and Technology—Written Assessment. http://www.publications.parliament.uk/pa/ld200203/ldselect/ldsctech/23/23w44.htm.

59. Keith Meldrum (MAFF CVO from 1988 to 1997), telephone interview, March 27, 2008.

60. UK Food Standards Agency. About Us. http://www.foodstandards.gov.uk/aboutus/.

61. John Roddick Russel MacGregor (Baron MacGregor of Pulham Market), telephone interview, May 14, 2008.

62. Van Zwanenberg and Millstone, BSE: Risk, Science, and Governance, 229–79.

63. The BSE Inquiry. Vol. 1: Findings and Conclusions. Was there a conflict of interest in MAFF. http://www.bseinquiry.gov.uk/report/volume1/chapt135.htm#647885.

64. There is a similar problem with the U.S. Food and Drug Administration. The same agency that approves drugs and is supported by the pharmaceutical industry also regulates the industry. There is an inherent conflict of interest, and as a result, postmarketing surveillance for adverse drug events receives far less support than the premarketing approval process. After a series of drug scandals, a crisis of confidence about FDA's performance led to a 2006 Institute of Medicine report, "The Future of Drug Safety: *Promoting and Protecting the Health of the Public.*" http://www.iom.edu/CMS/3793/26341/37329.aspx.

65. Sir Donald Acheson (chief medical officer of the UK Department of Health, 1983–91). personal communication, May 15, 2008.

66. *The BSE Inquiry.* Vol. 1: Findings and Conclusions. 13. What went right and what went wrong? Chief medical officers and chief veterinary officers. http://www.bseinquiry.gov.uk/report/volume1/chapt135.htm.

67. Federation of American Scientists, "Cost of Secrecy System Reaches Record High," *Secrecy News,* June 19, 2008. http://www.fas.org/blog/secrecy/2008/06/cost_of_secrecy.html.

68. P. Sanchez-Juan, S. N. Cousens, R. G. Will, and C. M. van Duijn, "Source of Variant Creutzfeldt-Jakob Disease Outside the United Kingdom," *Emerging Infectious Diseases* 13 (2007): 1166–69. http://www.cdc.gov/eid/content/13/8/1166.htm.

CHAPTER 7: THE VITAL LINK BETWEEN ANIMAL AND HUMAN HEALTH, PART II

1. Office Internationale des Epizootie. Foot and Mouth Disease. http://www.oie.int/eng/maladies/fiches/A_A010.hTM.

2. P. Gibbs, "The Foot-and-Mouth Disease Epidemic of 2001 in the U.K.: Implications for the USA and the 'War on Terror,'" *Journal of Veterinary Medical Education* 30 (2003): 121–32.

3. M. E. J. Woolhouse, "Foot-and-Mouth Disease in the U.K.: What Should We Do Next Time?" *Journal of Applied Microbiology* 94 (2003): 126S–130S.

4. *Foot and Mouth Disease: Lessons to Be Learned,* Inquiry Report HC888. Section 7: Silent Spread. http://archive.cabinetoffice.gov.uk/fmd/fmd_report/report/SECT_7.PDF.

5. D. Hemadri, C. Tosh, A. Sanyal et al., "Emergence of a New Strain of Type O Foot-and-Mouth Disease Virus: Its Phylogenetic and Evolutionary Relationship with the PanAsia Pandemic Strain," *Virus Genes* 25 (2002): 23–34.

6. *Foot and Mouth Disease: Lessons to Be Learned.*

7. Ibid. Section 5: Background to the 2001 Epidemic. http://archive.cabinetoffice.gov.uk/fmd/fmd_report/report/SECT_5.PDF.

8. *The Northumberland Report of 1968/9.* http://www.warmwell.com/northum.html).

9. *Foot and Mouth Disease: Lessons to Be Learned,* Section 5: Background to the 2001 Epidemic.

10. Ibid.

11. Ibid.

12. H. Rumbelow, "Deadly Virus That Blows in the Wind—Foot-and-Mouth," *London Times,* February 22, 2001.

13. *Foot and Mouth Disease: Lessons to Be Learned,* Section 8: The Immediate Response. http://archive.cabinetoffice.gov.uk/fmd/fmd_report/report/SECT_8. PDF).

14. Ibid.

15. H. Studd, "H. Foot-and-Mouth at Essex Farm Complex," *London Times,* February 21, 2001. See also H. Rumbelow, "Farmers Quarantined in Homes During Tests—Foot-and-Mouth," *London Times,* February 22, 2001.

16. Ibid.

17. *London Times,* "Stay at Home," February 24, 2001.

18. A. Norfolk, "Dirty Farm May Have Aided Virus—Foot-and-Mouth," *London Times,* February 24, 2001.

19. V. Elliott and H. Rumbelow, "Vets Say They Are Close to Source of Disease–Foot-and-Mouth," *London Times,* February 23, 2001.

20. P. Wilkinson, "Farmer Denies He Knew Pigs Were Infected—Foot-and-Mouth," *London Times,* February 24, 2001.

21. I. Cobain and H. Studd, "Farmer's Bid to Save 41p May Have Started It—Foot-and-Mouth Outbreak," *London Times,* March 28, 2001.

22. V. Elliott and P. Webster P. "Smuggled Meat Blamed for Epidemic—Foot-and-Mouth Outbreak," *London Times,* March 27, 2001.

23. V. Elliott, "Symptoms in Sheep Are Harder to Spot—Foot-and-Mouth," *London Times,* February 26, 2001.

24. V. Elliott, "Pounds 900 Sale of 18 Sheep Led to Rapid Outbreak," *London Times,* February 27, 2001. See also *Foot and Mouth Disease: Lessons to Be Learned,* Section 7. Silent Spread.

25. Ibid.

26. V. Elliott, "Outbreak Triggers Food-Chain Scrutiny—Foot-and-Mouth," *London Times,* February 24, 2001.

27. A. Sage, "French Praise Quick Action by the British—Foot-and-Mouth," *London Times,* February 26, 2001. See also *London Times,* "France Decided to Slaughter 30,000 Sheep—Foot-and-Mouth," March 1, 2001.

28. Elliott and Rumbelow, "Vets Say They Are Close to Source of Disease—Foot-and-Mouth."

29. M. Henderson, "Vets More Confident of Halting Outbreak—Foot-and-Mouth," *London Times,* March 7, 2001.

30. *Foot and Mouth Disease: Lessons to Be Learned,* Section 10: Pre-Emptive Slaughter. http://archive.cabinetoffice.gov.uk/fmd/fmd_report/report/SECT_10. PDF.

31. V. Elliott, "Badminton Horse Trials Cancelled—Foot-And-Mouth Outbreak," *London Times,* March 10, 2001.

32. *Foot and Mouth Disease: Lessons to Be Learned,* Section 10: Pre-Emptive Slaughter. See also M. Henderson, "Under Control? That Depends on How You Look at It—Foot-and-Mouth Outbreak," *London Times,* March 14, 2001.

33. Scottish Executive was the name of the Scottish government when it was formed in 1999. http://www.scotland.gov.uk/About/.

34. *Foot and Mouth Disease: Lessons to Be Learned,* Section 10: Pre-Emptive Slaughter.

35. *London Times,* "Silent Spring—Farming Needs Steady Hands Now and Brave Thinking Later," March 14, 2001.

36. *Herald and Sunday Herald* (Glasgow), "One Million Animals Must Die: Sentence Passed on Health Flocks in Bid to Isolate Rampaging Disease," March 16, 2001.

37. D. McGrory, "Suicide Fears over Isolated Farmers—Foot-and-Mouth Outbreak," *London Times,* March 15, 2001.

38. A. Pierce and V. Elliott, "Prince Gives Pounds 500,000 to Help Farmers—Foot-and-Mouth Outbreak," *London Times,* March 15, 2001.

39. R. Jenkins and V. Elliott, "No Reprieve for Sheep as Troops Prepare to Go In—Foot-and-Mouth Outbreak," *London Times,* March 20, 2001.

40. V. Elliott, "Farmers Protest at Delays and Red Tape Errors—Foot-and-Mouth Outbreak," *London Times,* March 20, 2001.

41. Jenkins and Elliott, "No Reprieve for Sheep."

42. *Foot and Mouth Disease: Lessons to Be Learned,* Section 10: Pre-Emptive Slaughter.

43. V. Elliott, "Outbreak Could Peak on May 3—Foot-and-Mouth Outbreak," *London Times,* March 22, 2001.

44. J. Sherman and V. Elliot, "Cabinet 'War Room' Pressed into Service—Foot-and-Mouth Outbreak," *London Times,* March 27, 2001.

45. A. Norfolk and P. Webster, "No 10 in Disarray over Vet Shortage." *London Times,* March 29, 2001.

46. Editorial, "Institutional Cull—MAFF Should Not Survive the Foot-and-Mouth Debacle," *London Times,* March 26, 2001.

47. V. Elliott and P. Webster, "Smuggled Meat Blamed for Epidemic—Foot-and-Mouth Outbreak," *London Times,* March 27, 2001.

48. *London Times,* "Foot and MAFF—What the Army Can Do for the Country Campaign," April 4, 2001.

49. *Foot and Mouth Disease: Lessons to Be Learned.* Section 10: Pre-Emptive Slaughter.

50. T. Reid, "Army Accuses Farmers of Infecting Their Own Animals," *London Times.* April 11, 2001.

51. T. Reid, "Vets in Open Revolt on 'Needless Slaughter,'" *London Times,* April 19, 2001.

52. M. Linklater, "Why Didn't Ministers Turn to the Real Expert?" *London Times,* April 26, 2001.

53. V. Elliott, "U-Turn on Cull Policy Saves Phoenix—Foot-and-Mouth Outbreak," *London Times,* April 26, 2001.

54. Gibbs, "The Foot-and-Mouth Disease Epidemic of 2001 in the U.K."

55. *Foot and Mouth Disease: Lessons to Be Learned,* Section 14: The Economic Impact of FMD. http://archive.cabinetoffice.gov.uk/fmd/fmd_report/report/SECT_14.PDF.

56. M. Mort, I. Convery, J. Baxter J et al., "Psychosocial Effects of the 2001 U.K. Foot and Mouth Disease Epidemic in a Rural Population: Qualitative Diary Based Study," *British Medical Journal* 331 (2005). http://www.bmj.com/cgi/content/full/331/7527/1234.

57. D.F. Peck, "Foot and Mouth Outbreak: Lessons for Mental Health Services," *Advances in Psychiatric Treatment* 11 (2005): 270–76.

58. M.H. Spooner, "Disease in Animals, Suicide in Humans," *Canadian Medical Association Journal* 169 (2003): 329. See also C. Booker and R. North, "How the Foot and Mouth Disaster of 2001 Began," *Sunday Telegraph* [London], August 12, 2001, 22.

59. Peck, "Foot and Mouth Outbreak."

60. Paul Kitching (former director of the World Reference Laboratory at the Institute for Animal Health; currently chief veterinary officer for Province of British Columbia, Canada), telephone interview, May 29, 2008.

61. Lord John Richard Krebs (principal of Jesus College, Oxford University and first chairman of the British Food Standards Agency), telephone interview, June 10, 2008.

62. In 2001, the Institute for Animal Health was composed of three laboratories: Compton, Pirbright, and the Neuropathogenesis Unit at Edinburgh University.

63. Prof. Donaldson defined dangerous contact premises (DC) as those identified by local investigations to have epidemiological links with infected premises (IP). The links could be a history of contact among animals between the IP and DC across a fence, movement of animals, vehicles (e.g., milk tankers), and so on from the IP to the DC during a period when animals on the IP would have been shedding virus. The usual procedure is to take a period of at least 14 to 21 days before disease was confirmed on the IP and to trace back any movements. If a premise is identified as a DC, the actions taken would depend on the risk assessment. If the risk is considered high, then the cloven-hoofed animals present would probably be culled. This is the traditional policy for FMD control and differs from what was done in 2001 in that it is based on an epidemiologic investigation and local knowledge. In contrast, under the 48-hour culling policy, when an IP was identified—even by clinical examination only (i.e., without laboratory confirmation), the neighboring premises (an average of five) would be assumed to be infected even though the boundaries between the IP and the contiguous premise were often poorly defined, and the animals on the IP were far away from those on the contiguous premises.

64. Professor Alex Donaldson (head of Pirbright Laboratory in 2001), telephone interview, June 12, 2008.

65. Centers for Disease Control and Prevention. Description of Viral Diseases: Hand-foot-mouth disease. http://www.cdc.gov/ncidod/dvrd/revb/enterovirus/hfhf.htm.

66. Dr. Joseph F. Annelli (Scientific and Technical Advisor for Emergency Management, APHIS, USDA), telephone interview, June 25, 2008. The opinions he expresses are his own and not those of USDA.

67. Sir Roy Anderson (FRS, FMedSci, rector of Imperial College London and professor of infectious disease epidemiology, Division of Epidemiology, Public Health and Primary Care), telephone interview, July 28, 2008.

68. Isabelle Chmitelin (DVM, chief veterinary officer, France, during 2001 FMD crisis), telephone interview, May 29, 2008.

69. A. McConnell and A. Stark, "Foot-and-Mouth 2001: The Politics of Crisis Management," *Parliamentary Affairs* 55 (2002): 664–81.

70. Ibid.

71. K. E. Jones, N. G. Patel, M. A. Levy et al., "Global Trends in Emerging Infectious Diseases," *Nature* 451 (2008): 990–94.

72. L. H. Kahn, B. Kaplan, T. P. Monath et al., "Teaching 'One Medicine, One Health,'" *The American Journal of Medicine* 121 (2008): 169–70.

CHAPTER 8: REACHING THE MASSES

1. U.S. Department of Health and Human Services, "Risk Communications During a Terrorist Attack or Other Public Health Emergency." http://www.hhs.gov/emergency.

2. P. Slovic, "Perception of Risk," *Science* 236 (1987): 280–85.

3. Ibid.

4. D. Holing, "It's the Outrage, Stupid," *Tomorrow,* March–April 1996. http://www.psandman.com/articles/holing.htm.

5. Slovic, "Perception of Risk."

6. Ibid.

7. E. Aakko, "Risk Communication, Risk Perception, and Public Health," *Wisconsin Medical Journal* 103 (2004): 25–27. In 1980, Congress established the Superfund program in cooperation with states after people became outraged at their exposure to toxic chemicals that were dumped into the ground and water. The Superfund program's mission is to locate, investigate, and clean up the worst hazardous waste dumps nationwide. http://www.epa.gov/superfund/about.htm.

8. Ibid.

9. G. M. Gray and D. P. Ropeik, "Dealing with the Dangers of Fear: The Role of Risk Communication," *Health Affairs* 21 (2002): 106–16.

10. L. K. Altman and G. Kolata, "Anthrax Missteps Offer Guide to Fight Next Bioterror Battle," *New York Times,* January 6, 2002.

11. Ibid.

12. U.S. Department of Health and Human Services, "Jeffrey P. Koplan, M.D., M.P.H." http://www.surgeongeneral.gov/library/youthviolence/koplan.htm. See also R. Pear, "Embattled Disease Agency Chief Is Quitting," *New York Times,* February 22, 2002.

13. J. P. Koplan, "Communication During Public Health Emergencies," *Journal of Health Communication* 8 (2003): 144–45.

14. Ibid.

15. B. Reynolds and M. W. Seeger, "Crisis and Emergency Risk Communication as an Integrative Model," *Journal of Health Communication* 10 (2005): 43–55.

16. Ibid.

17. National Research Council, *Improving Risk Communication* (Washington, DC: National Academy Press, 1989).

18. I. Weinstein, "An Outbreak of Smallpox in New York City," *American Journal of Public Health* 37 (1947): 1376–84.

19. J. W. Leavitt, "Be Safe. Be Sure: New York City's Experience with Epidemic Smallpox," *Hives of Sickness,* ed. D. Rosner (New Brunswick, NJ: Rutgers University Press, 1995).

20. Weinstein, "An Outbreak of Smallpox in New York City."

21. B. Roueche, "The Case of the Man from Mexico," *The New Yorker,* June 11, 1949, 70–83.

22. Ibid.

23. Ibid.

24. Leavitt, "Be Safe. Be Sure."

25. M. Lehman, "Smallpox. The Killer That Stalked New York," *Cosmopolitan,* April 1948.

26. *New York Times,* "Israel Weinstein: City's Health Chief" [Obituary], May 29, 1975.

27. *World-Telegram,* "Smallpox Kills 1, Infects 2 in City," April 4, 1947; and *New York Post,* "Smallpox Outbreak Kills 1.3 Cases Are First Caught Here in 25 Years," April 4, 1947.

28. Lehman, "Smallpox. The Killer That Stalked New York."

29. Roueche, "The Case of the Man from Mexico."

30. K. Pretshold and C. C. Sulzer, "Speed, Action and Candor. The Public Relations Story of New York's Smallpox Emergency," *Channels* 25 (1947, September): 3–6.

31. Ibid.

32. Leavitt, "Be Safe. Be Sure."

33. Roueche, "The Case of the Man from Mexico."

34. *New York Times,* "Second Smallpox Death Spurs Vaccination," April 13, 1947, 1.

35. Pretshold and Sulzer, "Speed, Action, and Candor."

36. Ibid.

37. Weinstein, "An Outbreak of Smallpox in New York City."

38. Pretshold and Sulzer, "Speed, Action, and Candor." See also *World Telegram,* "Vaccine Low, Mayor Calls Hurried Parley. Army, Navy and Drug Chiefs Asked to Join Smallpox Conference," April 15, 1947.

39. Leavitt, "Smallpox. The Killer That Stalked New York."

40. Weinstein, "An Outbreak of Smallpox in New York City."

41. *New York Times,* "Smallpox Danger Considered Past. Weinstein Tells Mayor Prompt Vaccination of 6,350,000 Averted Epidemic Here," May 12, 1947.

42. Weinstein, "An Outbreak of Smallpox in New York City."

43. Pretshold and Sulzer, "Speed, Action, and Candor."

44. J. W. Leavitt, "Public Resistance or Cooperation? A Tale of Smallpox in Two Cities," *Biosecurity and Bioterrorism* 1 (2003): 185–92.

45. Ibid.

46. B. Reynolds and M. W. Seeger, "Crisis and Emergency Risk Communication as an Integrative Model," *Journal of Health Communication* 10 (2005): 43–55.

47. K. Fearn-Banks, *Crisis Communications: A Casebook Approach* (Mahwah, NJ: Lawrence Erlbaum Assoc., 2002), 48–51.

48. Ibid.

49. F. Rowan, "Participation and Risk Communication," *International Journal of Emergency Mental Health* 4 (2002): 253–58.

50. C. Levy, "The Twitter Pandemic: Swine Flu Defines Social Media's New Age," *T.G. Daily,* April 28, 2009. http://www.tgdaily.com/content/view/42206/114/.

51. L. H. Kahn, "Stirring up "Swine Flu" Hysteria," *Bulletin of the Atomic Scientists,* May 11, 2009. http://www.thebulletin.org/web-edition/columnists/laura-h-kahn/stirring-swine-flu-hysteria; See also, http://twitter.com/CDCemergency.

52. Mark Perkiss (former reporter with the *Trenton Times;* currently spokesperson with New Jersey State Treasury), telephone interview, April 20, 2007.

53. Bill Jobes (director of news and public affairs, New Jersey Network News), telephone interview, May 10, 2007.

54. Donald Behm (reporter at *Milwaukee Journal Sentinel*), telephone interview, April 23, 2007.

55. In Canada's parliamentary system, the provincial ministers are elected positions. Tony Clement was elected to serve as the health minister of the Ontario province.

56. Andre Picard, Public Health Reporter, The *Globe and Mail,* telephone interview May 2, 2007.

57. Maureen Taylor, national health/medical reporter for CBC Television News, telephone interview May 11, 2007.

58. Donald A. Henderson (MD, MPH; Johns Hopkins Distinguished Service Professor and dean emeritus; professor of medicine and public health, University of Pittsburgh School of Medicine), telephone interview July 24, 2007.

59. K. Golan, "Surviving a Public Health Crisis: Tips for Communicators," *Journal of Health Communication* 8 (2003): 126–27.

60. E. Gursky, T. V. Inglesby, and T. O'Toole, "Anthrax 2001: Observations on the Medical and Public Health Response," *Biosecurity and Bioterrorism* 1 (2003): 97–110.

61. Ibid.

62. V. S. Freimuth, "Order Out of Chaos: The Self-Organization of Communication Following the Anthrax Attacks," *Health Communication* 20 (2006): 141–48.

63. Ibid.

64. Ibid.

65. Donald E. Low (MD, FRCPC; microbiologist in chief, Department of Microbiology, Mount Sinai Hospital, Toronto), telephone interview, May 29, 2007.

66. Richard Schabas (MD; chief of staff, York Central Hospital, Richmond Hill, Ontario, and Ontario chief medical officer of health from 1987 to 1997), telephone interview, May 31, 2007.

67. Low, telephone interview, May 29, 2007.

68. "The four horsemen" refers to the four physicians who ran the daily press conferences.

69. Schabas, telephone interview, May 31, 2007.

70. D. Drache and S. Feldman, "Media Coverage of the 2003 Toronto SARS Outbreak. A Report on the Role of the Press in a Public Crisis," Robarts Centre for Canadian Studies, York University, Toronto. http://www.yorku.ca/robarts/projects/global/papers/gcf_mediacoverageSARSto.pdf.

71. Ibid.

72. Drache and Feldman, "Media Coverage of the 2003 Toronto SARS Outbreak."

73. Ibid.

74. R. J. Griffin, S. Dunwoody, and F. Zabala, "Public Reliance on Risk Communication Channels in the Wake of a Cryptosporidium Outbreak," *Risk Analysis* 18 (1998): 367–75.

75. J. Browne, "Water Crisis Leaves Lingering Distrust," *Milwaukee Journal,* March 28, 1994, A4.

76. Griffin, Dunwoody, and Zabala, "Public Reliance on Risk Communication Channels."

77. Drache and Feldman, "Media Coverage of the 2003 Toronto SARS Outbreak."

CHAPTER 9: ALL HANDS ON DECK

1. Federal Emergency Management Agency, National Incident Management System (NIMS) resource center. http://www.fema.gov/emergency/nims/.

2. J. G. Hodge Jr., L. O. Gostin, K. Gebbie et al., "Transforming Public Health Law: The Turning Point Model State Public Health Act," *Journal of Law, Medicine, and Ethics* 34 (2006): 77–84.

3. L. O. Gostin, S. Burris, and Z. Lazzarini, "The Law and the Public's Health: A Study of Infectious Disease Law in the United States," *Columbia Law Review* 99 (1999): 59–128.

4. Institute of Medicine, *The Future of Public Health* (Washington DC: National Academy Press, 1988), 146.

5. G. J. Annas, "Bioterrorism, Public Health, and Civil Liberties," *New England Journal of Medicine* 346 (2002): 1337–42. See also Hodge, Gostin, Gebbie et al., "Transforming Public Health Law."

6. L. O. Gostin and J. G. Hodge Jr., *Turning Point. Collaborating for a New Century in Public Health* (University of Washington: Turning Point National Program Office, 2002), 31–34. http://www.turningpointprogram.org/Pages/pdfs/statute_mod/phsm_state_ph_law_assessment_report.pdf.

7. D. P. Fidler, "The Malevolent Use of Microbes and the Rule of Law: Legal

Challenges Presented by Bioterrorism," *Clinical Infectious Diseases* 33 (2001): 686–89.

8. U.S. Department of Justice, Presidential Decision Directive 39. http://www. ojp.usdoj.gov/odp/docs/pdd39.htm.

9. J.C. Butler, M.L. Cohen, C.R. Friedman et al., "Collaboration Between Public Health and Law Enforcement: New Paradigms and Partnerships for Bioterrorism Planning and Response," *Emerging Infectious Diseases* 8 (2002): 1152–56. http://www.cdc.gov/ncidod/eid/vol8no10/02-0400.htm. See also R.E. Hoffman and J.E. Norton, "Lessons Learned from a Full-Scale Bioterrorism Exercise," *Emerging Infectious Diseases* 6 (2000): 652–53.

10. Association of State and Territorial Health Officials (ASTHO), "Top 10 Suggestions from State Health Officials Who've Been There." http://www.astho. org/templates/display_pub.php?pub_id=323.

11. James W. Collins (Hamilton Township, New Jersey, police chief), telephone interview, June 14, 2007.

12. Kevin Hayden (formerly with New Jersey State Police), personal interview, July 23, 2007.

13. Kenneth Shuey (former FBI special agent; currently director of security, investigation, and internal audit, New Jersey Department of Motor Vehicles), telephone interview, June 15, 2007.

14. J. Warrick, "Trail of Odd Anthrax Cells Led FBI to Army Scientist," *Washington Post,* October 27, 2008, A01. http://www.washingtonpost.com/wp-dyn/content/article/2008/10/26/AR2008102602522.html.

15. Public Health Accreditation Board. http://www.phaboard.org/. See also E.S. Carpenter, "Is Public Health Credentialing Necessary?" *American Journal of Public Health* 85 (1995): 1712–13.

16. L.H. Kahn, "A Comparative Study of Four States' Public Health Systems: Survey Results from Local Health Departments, Physicians and Veterinarians." Final report to the Josiah Macy, Jr. Foundation, August 2006. http://www.princeton. edu/sgs/publications/Macy-Report_8-30-06_final.pdf.

17. Centers for Disease Control and Prevention, Career Epidemiology Career Field Officer Program. http://www.bt.cdc.gov/cotper/science/pdf/CEFO.pdf; See also http://www.bt.cdc.gov/cotper/science/cefo.asp.

18. Council of State and Territorial Epidemiologists, "2006 National Assessment of Epidemiologic Capacity: Findings and Recommendations." http://www. cste.org/pdffiles/2007/2006CSTEECAFINALFullDocument.pdf.

19. Federal Bureau of Investigation, "About Us—Quick Facts." http://www.fbi. gov/quickfacts.htm.

20. Environmental Protection Agency, "EPA History (1970–1985), Background: Why EPA Was Established." http://www.epa.gov/history/topics/epa/15b. htm.

21. Dr. Irwin Redlener (director of the National Center for Disaster Preparedness at Columbia University's Mailman School of Public Health and president of the Children's Health Fund), telephone interview, June 25, 2007.

22. Hanta virus, found in rodent urine or feces, caused a previously unrecognized

pulmonary disease in the American Southwest in 1993. Previously healthy young adults were getting sick and dying. See CDC *Morbidity and Mortality Weekly Report* 42 (1993): 816–20. http://www.cdc.gov/mmwr/preview/mmwrhtml/00030705. htm.

23. Dr. Ruth Berkelman (Rollins Chair and Director of the Center for Public Health Preparedness and Research at the Rollins School of Public Health at Emory University, Atlanta, Georgia; also deputy director of the National Center for Infectious Diseases of the CDC from 1992 to1997 and assistant surgeon general from 1995 to 2000), telephone interview, June 26, 2007.

24. L. H. Kahn and J. A. Barondess, "Preparing for Disaster: Response Matrices in the USA and UK," *Journal of Urban Health* 85 (2008): 910–22. 2008. http://www.springerlink.com/content/071751j49n00x637/.

25. Ibid.

26. FEMA National Response Framework (NRF) Resource Center. The NRF is a guide that details how the United States would conduct an all-hazards response to any type of crisis.

27. Mark Ghilarducci (vice president, James Lee Witt Associates), telephone interview, July 10, 2007.

28. L. M. Wein, "Neither Snow, Nor Rain, Nor Anthrax . . . ," *New York Times,* October 13, 2008. http://www.nytimes.com/2008/10/13/opinion/13wein.html? scp=4&sq=anthrax&st=cse.

29. Cornell University Law School, U.S. Code Collection, Title 10, Chapter 20, Section 401. http://www.law.cornell.edu/uscode/html/uscode10/usc_sec_10_ 00000401----000-.html.

30. C. T. Trebilcock, "The Myth of *Posse Comitatus,*" *Journal of Homeland Security* October 2000. http://www.homelandsecurity.org/journal/articles/Trebil cock.htm.

31. Federal Emergency Management Agency, Robert T. Stafford Disaster Relief and Emergency Assistance Act. http://www.fema.gov/pdf/about/stafford_act. pdf.

32. B. M. Lawlor, "Military Support of Civil Authorities—A New Focus for a New Millennium," *Journal of Homeland Security* October 2000 (updated September 2001). http://www.homelandsecurity.org/journal/Articles/Lawlor.htm.

33. U.S. Government Accountability Office, "Hurricane Katrina. Better Plans and Exercises Needed to Guide the Military's Response to Catastrophic Natural Disasters," GAO-06–808T, May 25, 2006. http://www.gao.gov/new.items/d06808t.pdf.

34. U.S. Government Accountability Office, "Bioterrorism: Public Health Response to Anthrax Incidents of 2001," October 2003. http://www.gao.gov/new. items/d04152.pdf. After the seven-year criminal investigation, circumstantial evidence pointed to one of the USAMRIID anthrax experts as the possible culprit behind the attacks. The troubled microbiologist took his own life before being charged with five counts of capital murder. See S. Shane and E. Lichtblau, "Scientist's Suicide Linked to Anthrax Inquiry," *New York Times,* August 2, 2008, A1. http://www.nytimes.com/2008/08/02/washington/02anthrax.html.

35. Federal Emergency Management Agency, Emergency Support Function Annexes: Introduction. http://www.fema.gov/pdf/emergency/nrf/nrf-esf-intro.pdf.

36. S. Izenberg, "Civilian Application of Military Resources," *Surgical Clinics of North America* 86 (2006): 665–73. See also Federal Emergency Management Agency, Emergency Support Function #8—Public Health and Medical Services Annex. http://www.fema.gov/pdf/emergency/nrf/nrf-esf-08.pdf.

37. The White House Homeland Security Presidential Directive/HSPD-5, Management of Domestic Incidents. http://www.dhs.gov/xabout/laws/gc_1214 592333605.shtm.

38. Federal Emergency Management Agency, Emergency Support Function #11—Agriculture and Natural Resources Annex. http://www.fema.gov/pdf/emer gency/nrf/nrf-esf-11.pdf.

39. Established in October 2002, the U.S. Northern Command (USNORTH-COM) is in charge of DOD homeland defense efforts and coordinates defense support of civil authorities. Its civil support mission includes disaster relief operations and managing the consequences of a terrorist attack. In most cases, the support would be limited, localized, and specific. USNORTHCOM has few permanently assigned forces. The *Posse Comitatus* Act prohibits military forces from becoming directly involved with law enforcement, but they can provide civil support in times of crisis such as a severe pandemic. http://www.northcom.mil/About/index.html.

40. Joseph M. Palma (MD, MPH, CPE.; retired acting deputy assistant to the secretary of defense for chemical/biological defense), telephone interview, May 31, 2007.

41. U.S. Army Medical Department Office of the Surgeon General, "Introduction to the U.S. Army Medical Department." http://www.armymedicine.army.mil/about/introduction.html.

42. U.S. Military Sealift Command, Ship Inventory. http://www.msc.navy.mil/inventory/inventory.asp?var=Hospitalship; and http://www.msc.navy.mil/factsheet/t-ah.htm.

43. S.W.A. Gunn, "Humanitarian, Noncombat Role for the Military," *Prehospital and Disaster Medicine* 9 (1994, Suppl. 2): S46–S48. See also United Nations Security Council Resolutions 1991, Resolution 688. http://daccessdds.un.org/doc/RESOLUTION/GEN/NR0/596/24/IMG/NR059624.pdf?OpenElement.

44. N. Joyce, "Civilian-Military Coordination in the Emergency Response in Indonesia," *Military Medicine* 171 (2006): 66–70.

45. Ibid.

46. S.F. McCartney, "Combined Support Force 536: Operation Unified Assistance," *Military Medicine* 171 (2006): 24–26.

47. Ibid.

48. D. Tarantino, "Asian Tsunami Relief: Department of Defense Public Health Response: Policy and Strategic Coordination Considerations," *Military Medicine* 171 (2006): 15–18.

49. L.C. Canas, K. Lohman, J.A. Pavlin et al., "The Department of Defense Laboratory-Based Global Influenza Surveillance System," *Military Medicine* 165 (2000, Supplement 2): 52–56.

50. U.S. Department of Defense, "Global Emerging Infections System," DoD-GEIS FY 2007 Annual Report, Executive Summary. http://www.geis.fhp.osd.mil/GEIS/aboutGEIS/annualreports/GEIS07AR.pdf.

51. DoD-GEIS Web About DoD-GEIS. http://www.geis.fhp.osd.mil/about GEIS.asp.

52. Institute of Medicine, *Review of the DoD-GEIS Influenza Programs: Strengthening Global Surveillance and Response.* 2007. National Academies Press. http://books.nap.edu/catalog.php?record_id=11974#toc.

53. Institute of Medicine, *Review of the DoD-GEIS Influenza Programs: Strengthening Global Surveillance and Response* (Washington, DC: National Academies Press, 2007). http://books.nap.edu/catalog.php?record_id=11974#toc.

CHAPTER 10: CONCLUSION

1. The "Dark Winter" scenario has been accused of choosing an extreme model for the spread of smallpox. M. Enserink, "How Devastating Would a Smallpox Attack Really Be?" *Science* May 2002; 296 (2002): 1592–95.

2. R. Pear, "Embattled Disease Agency Chief Is Quitting," *New York Times,* February 22, 2002.

3. J. W. Leavitt, "Public Resistance or Cooperation? A Tale of Smallpox in Two Cities," *Biosecurity and Bioterrorism* 1 (2003): 185–92.

4. R. Perez-Pena, "Web Sites That Dig for News Rise as Watchdogs," *New York Times,* November 18, 2008. http://www.nytimes.com/2008/11/18/business/media/18voice.html?hp.

5. L. Kahn, "Stirring up 'swine flu' hysteria," *Bulletin of the Atomic Scientists,* May 11, 2009. http://www.thebulletin.org/web-edition/columnists/laura-h-kahn/stirring-swine-flu-hysteria.

6. T. V. Inglesby, R. Grossman, and T. O'Toole, "A Plague on Your City: Observations from TOPOFF," *Clinical Infectious Diseases* 32 (2001): 436–45. See also T. O'Toole, M. Mair, and T. V. Inglesby, "Shining Light on 'Dark Winter,'" *Clinical Infectious Disease* 34 (2002): 972–83.

7. *New York Times,* "Fears May Be Outpacing Reality in Colorado Fires," June 16, 2002. http://www.nytimes.com/2002/06/16/us/fears-may-be-outpacing-reality-in-colorado-fires.html.

8. Andrew G. Flacks (U.S. Department of Health and Human Services/Office of Assistant Secretary for Preparedness and Response; liaison to Veterans Health Administration), telephone communication, February 24, 2009.

9. James D. Weed (director of homeland security and emergency management, National League of Cities), telephone communication, February 19, 2009.

INDEX

ABOUT THE AUTHOR

LAURA H. KAHN is a physician and research scholar in the Program on Science and Global Security at the Woodrow Wilson School of Public and International Affairs, Princeton University. Dr. Kahn writes monthly on-line columns on medicine, public health, and biosecurity issues for the *Bulletin of the Atomic Scientists* (http://www.thebulletin.org).